TABLE OF CONTENTS

Top 20 Test Taking Tips 1
Concepts of Kidney Disease 2
    Pathophysiology 2
    Measuring Kidney Function 16
    Complications 19
    Interventions 20
Hemodialysis 36
    Hemodialysis 41
    Complications 56
    Interventions 66
    Education 78
    Medication Administration 81
    Psychological and Sociocultural Interventions 85
    Infection Control 86
    Patient Rights and Regulatory Guidelines 92
Peritoneal Dialysis 95
    Peritoneal Dialysis Complications 100
    Interventions 103
Transplant 106
Acute Therapies 112
Practice Test 115
    Practice Questions 115
    Answers and Explanations 143
Secret Key #1 - Time is Your Greatest Enemy 169
    Pace Yourself 169
Secret Key #2 - Guessing is not Guesswork 169
    Monkeys Take the Test 169
    $5 Challenge 170
Secret Key #3 - Practice Smarter, Not Harder 171
    Success Strategy 171
Secret Key #4 - Prepare, Don't Procrastinate 171
Secret Key #5 - Test Yourself 172
General Strategies 172
Special Report: How to Overcome Test Anxiety 178
    Lack of Preparation 178
    Physical Signals 179
    Nervousness 179
    Study Steps 181
    Helpful Techniques 182
Additional Bonus Material 186

Top 20 Test Taking Tips

1. Carefully follow all the test registration procedures
2. Know the test directions, duration, topics, question types, how many questions
3. Setup a flexible study schedule at least 3-4 weeks before test day
4. Study during the time of day you are most alert, relaxed, and stress free
5. Maximize your learning style; visual learner use visual study aids, auditory learner use auditory study aids
6. Focus on your weakest knowledge base
7. Find a study partner to review with and help clarify questions
8. Practice, practice, practice
9. Get a good night's sleep; don't try to cram the night before the test
10. Eat a well balanced meal
11. Know the exact physical location of the testing site; drive the route to the site prior to test day
12. Bring a set of ear plugs; the testing center could be noisy
13. Wear comfortable, loose fitting, layered clothing to the testing center; prepare for it to be either cold or hot during the test
14. Bring at least 2 current forms of ID to the testing center
15. Arrive to the test early; be prepared to wait and be patient
16. Eliminate the obviously wrong answer choices, then guess the first remaining choice
17. Pace yourself; don't rush, but keep working and move on if you get stuck
18. Maintain a positive attitude even if the test is going poorly
19. Keep your first answer unless you are positive it is wrong
20. Check your work, don't make a careless mistake

Concepts of Kidney Disease

Pathophysiology

Functions of normal kidneys

Normal kidneys perform several functions including the following:
- Excretion of waste products of metabolism, including urea, uric acid, and water
- Maintenance of acid/base balance (pH)
- Regulation of plasma volume and blood pressure
- Maintenance of electrolyte balance
- Production (synthesis) of hormones, including erythropoietin (which stimulates erythrocyte production in response to low levels of O_2), renin (which regulates aldosterone), and calcitriol (which promotes the absorption of calcium)
- Reception of hormones, including antidiuretic hormone (ADH) produced by the pituitary, which enhances water reabsorption; aldosterone (from the adrenal cortex), which causes the kidneys to retain water and sodium (increasing the b/p); and parathyroid hormone (produced by the parathyroid glands), which increases the calcium: phosphate ratio and results in an increase in calcium in the blood.

Circulation of kidneys

The kidneys receive up to 25% of resting cardiac output. These highly vascular organs process an average of 1000 ml/min of blood. Circulation to each kidney begins with the renal artery, which branches from the abdominal aorta. The renal artery divides into interlobar arteries, which in turn supply the arcuate arteries. Interlobular arteries branch from the arcuates and further divide into afferent arterioles, which then become glomerular capillaries. The glomerular capillaries then merge to form efferent arterioles that disperse into vasa recta and peritubular capillaries.
- The vasa recta (straight arterioles) and their branches surround the loops of Henle of the juxtamedullary nephrons in the renal medulla, where they function to maintain the concentration gradient of the urine.
- The tiny peritubular capillaries lie adjacent to the nephrons permitting tubular secretion and reabsorption to take place.

Chronic kidney disease

According to the National Kidney Foundation, chronic kidney disease is defined as those patients with glomerular filtration rates of less than 60 ml/min/1.73 m^2 for greater than 3 months. The reasoning behind this is that at a GFR of less than 60, approximately half of the nephrons have been damaged. This is also the GFR where manifestations of chronic kidney disease begin to manifest including anemia, early bone disease, and establishes an increased risk for coronary artery disease.

Stages
The five stages of chronic kidney disease are listed and defined below:
- Stage I—Glomerular filtration rate > 90 ml/min/1.73 m^2
- Stage II—Glomerular filtration rate between 60 – 90 ml/min/1.73 m^2
- Stage III—Glomerular filtration rate between 30 – 60 ml/min/1.73 m^2
- Stage IV—Glomerular filtration rate between 15 – 30 ml/min/1.73 m^2
- Stage V—Glomerular filtration rate <15 ml/min/1.73 m^2 (needs dialysis)

Screening
Screening for CKD is necessary for any patient considered in the high-risk category. Kidney function and an evaluation of proteinuria are both important in assessing a patient for CKD. Since diabetics are at high risk for developing CKD, the American Diabetes Association (ADA) recommends that all patients diagnosed with type 2 diabetes be tested for microalbuminuria at the time of diagnosis. Type 1 diabetics should be tested 5 years after the initial evaluation. Any patient with hypertension or heart disease or who is in any other high-risk group should have routine examinations for kidney involvement. The dipstick test for albumin and blood cells is the first step in analyzing the patient for kidney disease. If positive for albumin, the next step is a protein-creatinine ratio test. If the dipstick is positive for blood or white cells, a more comprehensive microscopic analysis needs to be done.

Risk factors
The major risk factors for chronic kidney disease include:
- diabetes mellitus
- hypertension
- hyperlipidemia
- smoking

These are preventable and very treatable causes of both initiating and progressing kidney disease. They are also the most widely prevalent and present the greatest risk to public health. Other less common risk factors include:
- autoimmune diseases (chiefly systemic lupus erythematosus)
- chronic urinary tract infections
- age, renal stones
- systemic infections
- family history

Polycystic kidney disease as a cause
Polycystic kidney disease is the most common genetic condition that can cause renal disease. It is usually inherited in an autosomal dominant fashion, though there are some recessive patterns of inheritance. The usual disease course is one where renal failure develops in young persons between 25-35 years of age. The only treatment is renal replacement therapy and most patients require transplants. It is characterized by large kidney sizes with huge cysts that can often be palpated on physical exam. There are no known treatments that can effectively slow the progression of the disease.

Metabolic acidosis
The kidneys are involved in excreting broken down proteins. Proteins break down into their component parts, which are amino acids. Amino acids are, in fact, acids. They are largely buffered in the bloodstream via the presence of the ubiquitous base bicarbonate. When renal failure ensues,

the ability to excrete amino acids is hindered. With amino acid build up, the bicarbonate buffer is also exhausted. Therefore, the amino acid build up contributes to the acidosis present in all patients with chronic kidney disease. Renal replacement therapy with appropriate dialysate solutions aids in eliminating the acidosis. Thus, before each dialysis treatment patients are acidotic. Following dialysis, patients should ideally return to neutrality or a pH of 7.4.

Effects on neurological system
Most patients suffer neurological consequences from chronic uremia. The uremic syndrome can cause dementia marked by incoherent speech, seizures and EEG changes. The precise etiology of uremia-induced dementia has yet to be elucidated. Another less common cause of dementia is chronic aluminum exposure. Aluminum has been shown to accumulate in patients with chronic kidney disease. The most common source of aluminum used to be phosphate binders. Although aluminum induced dementia is rare today, it is still seen with aluminum coming from contaminated water supplies. Another neurologic consequence of dialysis is neuropathy. The exact mechanism is unknown but the neuropathy presents as numbness or burning of the extremities, reduced vibratory sense and twitching. Inadequate dialysis has been implicated as a possible cause for the neuropathy but more research is needed.

Effects on joints
Patients on renal replacement therapy frequently have elevated uric acid levels. Uric acid is implicated in causing gout. Gout is a disease where uric acid crystals precipitate and deposit into joints. The most common joints involved include the distal joint of the great toe, elbows and knees. Another disease of the joints that is frequently seen in dialysis patients is pseudogout. Pseudogout is arthritis where calcium pyrophosphate crystals deposit into joints. Patients will complain of pain and inflammation at the wrist, fingers, back of the hands and knees. Finally, β2 microglobulin amyloidosis causes joint pains and hemarthrosis (blood in joints). It affects nearly any joint in the body.

Effects on reproductive endocrine system
Women on dialysis rarely menstruate if at all. The ability to ovulate has also come into question. Uremia seems to interfere with the normal hormonal balance and appears to quell ovulation. In men, uremia has been shown to decrease sperm production. Furthermore, libido in both sexes is markedly reduced. The exact etiology for the described endocrine phenomena is unknown. They seem to be another piece of the puzzle in the constellation of symptoms, which contribute to the uremic syndrome.

Effects on respiratory system
Patients with chronic kidney disease do not adequately excrete water. Thus, patients on dialysis are frequently volume overloaded. When the excess water is combined with weakened cardiac muscle, pulmonary edema occurs. Patients on dialysis frequently battle pulmonary edema and the best therapy is dialysis with increased filtration or transmembrane pressures. The elevated transmembrane pressure will forcibly push the excess water through the dialyzer under convective forces.

Effects on cardiovascular system
Chronic kidney disease is frequently associated with hypertension and fluid retention. Hypertension and fluid retention is taxing to the heart and can lead to myocardial wall thickening called left ventricular hypertrophy. Left ventricular hypertrophy is an increase in the size of the left ventricle secondary to increased stress placed on the heart from hypertension and excess fluid. Chronic left ventricular hypertrophy can lead to heart failure. Ace inhibitors are the drug of choice

in treating patients with left ventricular hypertrophy and those who have progressed to congestive heart failure. Other effects of renal failure on the cardiovascular system include coronary artery calcification and pericarditis. The heart is surrounded by a sac, which can become inflamed and fluid filled. When that happens, it is known as pericarditis. Pericarditis frequently presents as chest pain with a friction rub heard on auscultation. It is an indication for urgent dialysis.

Effects on gastrointestinal system
Patients with chronic kidney disease frequently complain of decreased appetite and metallic tastes in their mouths. Both are due to complications of uremia with little treatment options. Another common gastrointestinal issue is one of internal bleeding. The mucosa of the gastrointestinal tract is more friable because of the systems inability to coagulate (platelet dysfunction). Thus, patients on dialysis will frequently have gastrointestinal bleeding. Proton pump inhibitors are one measure to help aid in the healing of any gastric or peptic ulcers noted. Lower gastrointestinal bleeds may require colonoscopy or bowel resection depending on the extent of the bleeding.

Effects on integumentary system
Foremost, ecchymosis is frequently seen on the skin of most patients. This is due to a combination of frequent blood draws and platelet dysfunction. Also seen is skin pallor, which is secondary to anemia of chronic disease. Finally, patients with uremic syndrome symptoms may experience pruritus for reasons unknown. They will frequently itch and scars and erythema are frequently noted.

ESRD

Effects on immune system
In the early stages of the immune deficiency, uremic toxins are thought to play an important role while the dialysis procedure itself leads to a state of chronic inflammation. Infection is the second most common cause of death in ESRD patients with cardiovascular mortality ranking number one. Immunodepression contributes to the high incidence of infection in this group. The combination of reduced WBC count and poor granulocytic response to infection results in decreased bacteriocidal capability. Other contributing factors are malnutrition, frequency of cannulation, and invasive procedures. The elevated uremic level has an effect on the body's ability to develop a fever as a response to infection. The ESRD patient may present with a subnormal body temperature, so care must be taken to assess the patient's response to infection.

Effects on endocrine system
Endocrine system effects in the ESRD patients include the following:
- Insulin production
- Parathyroid hormone levels disorder
- Increased plasma norepinephrine
- Inconsistent epinephrine levels
- Increased aldosterone
- Elevated levels of glucagon (pancreatic hormone used for carbohydrate metabolism) and gastrin (stimulates the secretion of gastric acid), which occurs as a consequence of renal metabolism clearance
- Hypothyroidism
- Low response to thyroid-releasing hormone (TRH) with mostly normal response to thyroid-stimulating hormone (TSH)

- Increased growth hormone and prolactin
- Abnormal production of estrogen, progesterone, or testosterone
- Elevated luteinizing hormone (LH) in both sexes

Effects on hematologic system
The most common problem is anemia. Kidney failure leads to a decrease in erythropoietin production, which leads to less red blood cell production by the bone marrow. Anemia is treated with supplemental erythropoietin and iron. Another frequently encountered hematologic abnormality is platelet dysfunction. Platelets are important in clotting and help prevent excess blood loss. Yet, uremia alters platelet function and bleeding diathesis is problematic. Hemodialysis patients require frequent blood draws, which leaves them with bruising and hematomas. Moreover, gastrointestinal bleeding is concerning for the body is incapable of adequately quelling the loss of blood. Proton pump inhibitors aid in alleviating blood loss secondary to gastric ulcers.

Causes of chronic kidney disease in children

The most common causes of chronic kidney disease in children are congenital anomalies. These include:
- Obstructive uropathy
- Reflux nephropathy
- Renal dysplasia
- Autosomal recessive polycystic kidney disease
- Other hereditary diseases

Acquired forms of chronic kidney disease include glomerular diseases such as focal segmental glomerulosclerosis and membranoproliferative glomerulonephritis.

Prerenal failure

Pathophysiology
Prerenal failure is due to an inadequate blood pressure reaching the renal arteries. The renal arteries respond to low blood pressure by releasing the local hormone renin. Renin causes the release of angiotensin I which travels to the lungs and causes the release of the potent angiotensin II. Angiotensin II causes vasoconstriction of the renal arteries, which will help elevate the pressure delivered to the kidneys. It is important to know that ace inhibitors act to block the converting enzyme, which produces angiotensin II. While this may seem counterintuitive, it is important to differentiate the physiology of acute renal failure and normal renal function. Under normal physiologic conditions, ace inhibitors are helpful in preventing the progression of renal failure. However, during acute renal failure, ace inhibitors are contraindicated.

Major causes
Prerenal failure results from anything that causes decreased blood flow to the kidneys. This includes:
- Dehydration
- Congestive heart failure
- Liver cirrhosis
- Septic shock

- Cardiogenic shock
- Anaphylactic shock
- Medications

Dehydration results from excess intravascular water loss secondary to exercise, diarrhea, and vomiting. Congestive heart failure and liver cirrhosis deliver less blood volume to the kidneys. The former is due to an ineffective pump (the heart) and the latter is due to third spacing (fluids leaving the vascular system and entering the interstitium). Septic shock is found with blood born pathogens particularly gram-negative bacteria. Cardiogenic shock results when the heart is incapable of pumping blood effectively usually from an acute infarction. Anaphylactic shock is secondary to the release of histamines in response to an allergen. Medications causing prerenal failure include diuretics and ace inhibitors.

Congestive heart failure and dehydration: Congestive heart failure occurs when cardiac muscle fails to pump blood effectively. This can be due to either an inability of cardiac muscle to contract (systolic dysfunction) or relax (diastolic dysfunction). Both mechanisms lead to ineffective circulating blood volumes reaching the kidney.

Dehydration by any mechanism results in a loss of effective circulating volume. The major reasons for dehydration include:
- Exercise
- Diarrhea
- Vomiting
- Medications, chiefly diuretics

The effect of both instances is acute renal failure secondary to prerenal azotemia. The kidney responds by releasing renin, a local hormone which causes the release of angiotensin I. Angiotensin I travels to the lungs and is converted to angiotensin II which is a potent vasoconstrictor. Angiotensin II will cause the renal arteries to constrict and increase the blood pressure at the level of the kidneys.

Liver cirrhosis and septic shock: Liver cirrhosis is a very common cause of acute renal failure in patients with chronic liver disease. The mechanism is as follows: fluid accumulates in the interstitium and lower extremities due to the lack of serum albumin. The liver produces albumin. Albumin is the chief protein responsible for providing the oncotic pressure needed to retain fluid in the vascular system. Without albumin, fluid will traverse the blood vessels and enter the interstitium via osmosis.

Septic shock is caused by an overwhelming infection in the bloodstream, most commonly from gram negative bacteria. The immune system is overwhelmed by the infectious agent and the response is a loss of vasomotor tone. The arteries vasodilate to the point of causing hypotension. The decrease in blood pressure leads to an ineffective volume reaching the kidneys.

The effect of both conditions is acute renal failure secondary to prerenal azotemia.

Cardiogenic shock and anaphylactic shock: Cardiogenic shock is not unlike congestive heart failure in its mechanism for causing acute renal failure. Cardiogenic shock is due to a myocardium which does not pump effectively. However, unlike with congestive heart failure, cardiogenic shock is usually an acute event. The most common cause of cardiogenic shock is a large myocardial infarction. When the heart does not pump effectively, the systemic blood pressure falls and the kidneys sense this drop in pressure.

Anaphylactic shock is due to the body's response to an allergen. Unlike allergies causing nasal congestion or hives, this response is far more severe. The release of histamine from the body causes the blood vessels to vasodilate and results in hypotension. The hypotension causes a decrease in blood pressure at the level of the kidney. The effect of both conditions is acute renal failure secondary to prerenal azotemia.

Ace inhibitors: Ace inhibitors are commonly used to prevent the progression of renal disease in patients with chronic kidney disease. Their mechanism of action is such that they can also precipitate acute renal failure. When the kidney senses a decrease in blood pressure, it responds by releasing renin, a local hormone which causes the release of angiotensin I. Angiotensin I travels to the lungs and is converted to angiotensin II which is a potent vasoconstrictor. Angiotensin II will cause the renal arteries to constrict and increase the blood pressure at the level of the kidneys. Ace-inhibitors act by blocking the enzyme angiotensin converting enzyme. This enzyme is the key step in the conversion of angiotensin to angiotensin II. While ace-inhibitors have been effective in stopping proteinuria and progression of chronic kidney disease, they can also precipitate acute renal failure by the aforementioned mechanism.

Intrinsic renal failure

Intrinsic renal failure is secondary to directly injury to the renal parenchyma. Specifically, the damage can occur to the renal tubules, interstitium, glomeruli and renal arteries and veins. Damage that occurs to the interstitium includes those caused by medications, chiefly non-steroidal anti-inflammatory drugs and antibiotics (penicillins and aminoglycosides). The list of medications causing renal damage is too exhaustive to list but the most common include lithium, chemotherapies, heavy metals and amphotericin (antifungal). Glomerular damage is secondary to systemic lupus erythematosus, glomerulonephritis and various forms of vasculitis. Renal arteries and veins are damaged by embolic phenomena from atrial fibrillation and endocarditis. Other causes of intrinsic renal failure include ischemia and damage from radiocontrast administered during angiograms and cat scans.

Infections that can scar kidneys

An infection of the kidney and renal pelvis is termed pyelonephritis. This occurs when bacteria, usually from the bowel, ascend through the lower urinary tract. Once in the kidney, the infection may lead to fibrosis and scarring. Fluoroquinolones (ciprofloxacin), amoxicillin, cephalosporin, and trimethoprim are the drugs of choice for treatment of these infections. If leukocytosis and a high fever are present, IV administration of the antibiotic may be indicated. *Mycobacterium tuberculosis* cause renal tuberculosis as a secondary site to the primary lung infection. Caseation, in which dead tissue decays and forms a dry mass, occurs in the tubercular lesions. The kidneys are scarred, calcified, and permanently damaged. Findings may include dysuria, hematuria, sterile pyuria, albuminuria, and urgency. The client may complain of suprapubic pain, increased urination, and fever. Diagnosis is by culture of acid-fast bacillus, cystoscopy, needle biopsy, or imaging. Renal tuberculosis often remains dormant for several years after the patient's pulmonary infection before causing any symptoms.

Post renal failure

Post renal failure results when there is an obstruction of urinary flow out of the kidneys. The most common causes include prostatic hypertrophy, crystal disease and extrarenal causes of ureteral obstruction. When the prostate enlarges, it can block urinary flow as it passes through the urethra. Crystal disease includes kidney stones secondary to uric acid, calcium or struvite stones. The crystals deposit in the distal tubules of the kidney and cause tubular damage resulting in an inability to generate adequate urine flow. Extrarenal causes of ureteral obstruction include retroperitoneal fibrosis, bladder cancer and colon cancer (the tumor enlarges from the colon and compresses the urethra).

Infectious causes of renal failure

The most common infectious cause of renal failure is bacterial. Pyelonephritis is inflammation of the kidneys secondary to an infectious agent, usually bacterial. Treatment includes use of broad-spectrum antibiotics, usually quinolones. Other less common causes include mycobacterium tuberculosis and fungal infections. Both have been known to cause renal failure in immunocompromised patients and those with HIV. Finally, a rare but interesting cause of renal failure is post streptococcal glomerulonephritis. Patients will have strep throat and two weeks later present with renal failure and hematuria. The renal failure is caused by streptococcal antigens forming immune complexes that deposit in the glomerulus. This immune complex causes the glomerulonephritis and renal failure ensues. The renal failure is usually self-limited and patients recover full kidney function after approximately a two week course.

PKD

Polycystic kidney disease (PKD) is the third leading cause of renal failure. It is a genetic disease, and both sexes are equally likely to be affected. Dominant genes cause most cases of PKD with one rare type originating from a recessive gene. In the recessive gene type of PKD, the disease becomes symptomatic early in childhood and usually has a poor prognosis. In the more common form, the autosomal dominant, symptoms may present in early (50% develop cysts before age 18) to mid-adulthood. Fluid-filled cysts replace normal kidney tissue, as these cysts grow; they crowd the healthy tissue until kidney function deteriorates.

Symptoms may include the following:
1. Flank or low-back pain
2. Urinary tract infections
3. Hematuria
4. Severe hypertension
5. Fatigue
6. Nausea
7. Kidney stones with accompanying pain
8. Increase in abdominal girth Infection of the kidneys may further weaken the kidneys ability to function. Nephrectomy may be the only option for the painful, chronically infected kidney.

In addition to cysts in the kidneys, PKD may cause cysts to form in the liver, pancreas, testes, ovaries and spleen. Brain aneurysms have been found in approximately 10% of PKD cases.

Nephrotic syndrome

Nephrotic syndrome is a myriad of clinical findings that result in massive losses of protein through the kidney due to damaged, leaky glomeruli. When the protein level in the blood declines, fluid shifts into the tissues resulting in edema. Patients with nephrotic syndrome are at an increased risk for thrombosis and infection. Pitting edema in the legs, puffiness in the periorbital area upon awakening, abdominal ascites, and pulmonary edema may be seen with this syndrome. The high protein level may cause the urine to appear 'foamy'. Dietary recommendations include a low sodium diet, avoidance of saturated fats, monitoring of fluid intake, and increased fruits and vegetables. Treatment depends upon the underlying cause of the condition. Immunosuppressants, diabetic blood glucose control, and hypertension medications to maintain blood pressure levels are used to treat the underlying disease processes that lead to the nephrotic syndrome.

Nephrotic syndrome is defined by the following: heavy proteinuria (>3.5 gms over 24 hours), hyperlipidemia, hypercoagulability, edema with frequent hypertension. The edema is caused by the excessive protein loss in the urine. The lack of protein in the serum causes fluids to shift into the interstitial and intracellular spaces. Thus, patients with nephrotic syndrome retain a lot of fluid in dependent areas. It is caused by a myriad of conditions including diabetes, glomerulonephritis, lupus and hypertension. Treatment is targeted at treating the underlying condition with use of diuretics and ace inhibitors. The former is to relieve excess water retention and the latter is to slow the progression of protein loss and further kidney damage.

Amyloidosis

Amyloidosis is a rare disorder and is either primary or secondary. Primary amyloidosis is caused by deposition of light chains from antibodies. These proteins cause organ dysfunction and lead to renal failure. Primary amyloidosis carries a poor prognosis and treatments are not curative. Secondary amyloidosis is a more chronic and progressive condition where proteins deposit in most any organ system. Again, these proteins cause organ dysfunction and they can deposit in the heart, liver, skin and kidneys. Treatment options are also limited and renal failure is treated with replacement therapy. The only known agents to slow the progression of renal failure from amyloidosis are ace inhibitors.

Renal cell carcinoma

Renal cell carcinoma is cancer of the kidney as the name implies. It is usually diagnosed in patients over 50 who present with painless hematuria. Renal cell cancers also secrete erythropoietin. Thus, checking erythropoietin levels is a diagnostic clue. CAT scans and ultrasounds are used to locate the tumor and biopsies are performed to grade the cancer. Treatment consists of a nephrectomy with attempts to preserve the other kidney. However, if both kidneys are affected (rare), than bilateral nephrectomies are indicated. Renal replacement therapy is offered to those who require it.

Renal artery stenosis

Renal artery stenosis is a condition where there is a significant narrowing of the renal arteries. There are two primary causes:
- Fibromuscular dysplasia (more common in young women)
- Atherosclerosis

Fibromuscular dysplasia is caused by smooth muscle build up in the renal arteries causing a narrowing of the lumen. Atherosclerosis is the same mechanism of luminal narrowing as found in patients with coronary artery disease. Patients with renal artery stenosis present with severe hypertension and often develop renal failure (from a lack of adequate blood supply). Treatment includes stents and renal artery bypass surgery. Ace inhibitors are a relative contraindication in patients with renal artery stenosis.

Albumin

In ESRD patients, serum albumin levels are important in predicting morbidity and mortality. Albumin is the most prevalent protein found in plasma. It has the role of transporting the smaller molecules of drugs, calcium and bilirubin in the bloodstream. It helps maintain the fluid volume in the blood vessels. This form of protein is an accurate gauge for the nutritional status of the ESRD patient. The levels are a direct reflection of the diet protein intake, which may be insufficient due to the patient's lack of appetite. The desired range for serum albumin in the ESRD patient is greater than 4.0g/dL. Symptoms of low serum albumin (hypoalbuminemia) include edema, weight loss, muscle wasting, fatigue, and hypotension. The risks for morbidity and mortality increase as the serum albumin levels decrease, especially in patients where the level is less than 3.5g/dL.

Relationship between CRP and serum albumin levels

The body produces C-reactive protein (CRP) as a response to tissue trauma, infection, and inflammation. An elevation of more than 50mg/L is an accurate indicator of an acute inflammatory process in the dialysis patient. It may signal a retained failed allograft or a failed arteriovenous graft with undiagnosed infection. High CRP levels can be an indicator of mortality. CRP levels usually hit the highest level 2-3 days after an infection, increasing by as much as 100 times or more with a bacterial or viral infection. Within 1-2 weeks after the infection, the levels begin to drop. CRP values are useful in forecasting low serum albumin levels; evaluate any resistance to Epogen (epoetin alfa) therapy, evaluate the effectiveness of treatment of infections, and identify occult infections and chronic inflammation.

Potassium

Potassium is necessary for the normal functioning of the neuromuscular, skeletal, and cardiac systems as well as smooth muscle activity and intracellular enzyme responses. It is the most prevalent intracellular positively charged ion (cation) and the second most plentiful in the body. Acid base balance affects potassium levels in the cells. Hypokalemia refers to an abnormally low level of serum potassium (less than 3.5mEq). Causes of hypokalemia include vomiting and diarrhea, abuse of laxatives, anorexia nervosa, diuretics, excessive perspiration, burns, and diet insufficiency. Symptoms appear as weakness, fatigue, and arrhythmias.

Hyperkalemia

When the serum potassium level reaches 5.5mEq/L, the condition is hyperkalemia. Excessive intake of potassium-rich foods is the usual culprit, but crush injury, transfusions, catabolic states, GI bleeding, hemolysis, and acidosis are also possible causes. The patient may complain of shortness of breath, cramping, diarrhea, dizziness, and muscle weakness. Cardiac effects range from arrhythmias to cardiac arrest. A rapid change in the serum potassium levels significantly affects the symptoms. Kayexalate, sodium bicarbonate, glucose, and insulin may be administered to treat this condition, but the most effective treatment is dialysis. Dialysis patients on digoxin must be closely monitored for toxicity as serum potassium decreases.

Kidney's role in calcium and phosphorus homeostasis

The kidney is instrumental in excreting excess phosphorus and producing the active form of vitamin D, called calcitriol. Calcitriol is a hormone which travels to the gut and aids in both phosphorus and calcium absorption. Moreover, calcium and phosphorus are regulated by the hormone PTH (parathyroid hormone). PTH is released from the parathyroid gland and functions to elevate serum calcium levels and lower phosphorus levels. Note that the kidneys are involved in both phosphorus excretion (under influence of PTH) and phosphorus absorption via calcitriol.

Effects of renal failure on calcium and phosphorus levels

Renal failure causes a decrease in calcitriol production. Thus, there is lower calcium and phosphorus absorption taking place at the gut. The parathyroid gland senses the lower calcium levels and releases PTH. PTH attempts to raise calcium in the blood but also attempts to excrete excess phosphorus via the kidney. However, kidney function is subnormal and phosphorus is not excreted appropriately. The end result of renal failure is phosphorus accumulation and subnormal calcium levels. The reservoir for the body's calcium is bone. With PTH levels elevated to compensate for the lack of calcium absorption, bone disease ensues. The calcium is taken from bone and released into the bloodstream in response to PTH's stimulation. Interventions to bind phosphate in the gut and elevate serum calcium through oral vitamin D are needed in patients with chronic kidney disease.

Role of PTH on calcium and phosphorus

Parathyroid hormone (PTH) is stimulated by two mechanisms: either a low serum calcium level or elevated phosphorus. PTH acts to increase serum calcium and lower phosphorus. It increases calcium by two methods.
- The first is to stimulate the release of calcium from bone (the body's reservoir of calcium stores).
- The second is to stimulate the kidney to release calcitriol, the active form of Vitamin D. Calcitriol will raise serum calcium levels by increasing calcium absorption at the gut.

Finally, PTH acts to decrease serum phosphorus. It accomplishes this by acting on the kidneys to excrete phosphorus in the urine. In patients with chronic kidney disease, PTH is elevated because the kidneys do not respond appropriately. The kidneys can neither produce calcitriol nor excrete phosphorus. Thus, PTH levels rise (also known as secondary hyperparathyroidism) and a viscous cycle ensues.

Importance of calcium-phosphorus product

When the calcium and phosphorus levels reach a certain point, they can combine in the bloodstream and precipitate out. They form mineral deposits in organs as well as blood vessels, which is injurious to their function. Thus, nephrologists must keep track of the calcium-phosphorus product or simply multiply the serum calcium with the serum phosphorus. If the product exceeds 70, the patient is at increased risk of calcium-phosphorus deposition. Therefore, it is imperative to monitor the calcium-phosphorus product in all patients with chronic kidney disease with interventions to lower that product if necessary.

Renal Bone Disease: Renal osteodystrophy

Renal osteodystrophy is a general term that includes many aspects of renal bone disease. It includes:
- Osteitis fibrosa cystica
- Osteomalacia
- Adynamic bone disease
- Mixed osteodystrophy

Briefly, osteitis fibrosa cystica exists when there is increased bone turnover from elevated PTH (hyperparathyroidism). Osteomalacia occurs when there is low bone turnover in combination with aluminum deposition. Adynamic bone disease occurs when bone turnover is low secondary to reduced parathyroid hormone. Finally, mixed osteodystrophy exists when there is a mixture of both high and low bone turnover. Again, renal osteodystrophy is a general term that encompasses all of the aforementioned entities.

Osteitis fibrosa cystica

Osteitis fibrosa cystica is the term used to define excess bone turnover in response to both elevated PTH (hyperparathyroidism) and low calcitriol. The driving force behind this response is elevated phosphorus levels and low calcium. The elevation in PTH causes calcium to be released from bone resulting in what is termed increased bone turnover. Increased bone turnover results in weakened bone structure and an osteoporosis of sorts. This leads towards an increased susceptibility to fractures (the most worrisome being hip fractures). Correction of increased bone turnover and thus osteitis fibrosa cystica is through administration of phosphate binders, consumption of low phosphorus diets, and supplementation of calcitriol.

Osteomalacia

Osteomalacia is defined by low bone turnover secondary to aluminum deposition. In the past, efforts to decrease phosphorus were done with the use of aluminum binders. Aluminum was very good at binding phosphorus in the gut and thus preventing its absorption. Unfortunately, aluminum has some serious side effects. One side effect is that it deposits into bone and replaces the normal bony matrix. Thus, parathyroid hormone will act on bone, which is devoid of normal calcium and will be chronically elevated. This entity has largely vanished with the use of newer phosphate binders that do not use aluminum.

Adynamic bone disease

Adynamic bone disease occurs when bone turnover is absent. The pathophysiology is as follows: parathyroid hormone levels are increased in response to low serum calcium and renal failure. Therapy is begun with calcium containing phosphate binders and calcitriol. The resulting increase in calcium and lowering of phosphorus causes PTH levels to decrease to near normal levels. This causes bone to be essentially dormant. The physiology of a patient with chronic kidney disease dictates that PTH levels at 1.5 – 2 times normal are needed in order to maintain healthy bone turnover. Otherwise, bone becomes dormant and essentially inactive. Thus, when treating patients for hyperphosphatemia and vitamin D deficiency, care must be taken not to be overzealous so as not to reduce PTH levels to normal.

Effects of metabolic acidosis on normal bone homeostasis

Metabolic acidosis contributes to renal bone disease by causing the release of calcium from bone. In patients with chronic kidney disease, amino acids are not readily excreted and the acids accumulate. The normal buffer for acids is bicarbonate. When the bicarbonate is exhausted, bone serves as a buffer. In acting as a buffer, bone releases calcium while absorbing the acids. Thus, bone is devoid of its vital elements making it weaker and more susceptible to fractures.

Correction of the acidosis will allow for the proper buffering of acids and allow calcium to remain in the bony matrix.

Calciphylaxis

Calciphylaxis is a rare complication of metastatic calcification. It occurs when the calcium-phosphorus product is high. Calcium precipitates in arteries and tissues including vital organs and skin. In contrast to metastatic calcification, calciphylaxis causes tissue ischemia. Patients frequently present with gangrenous skin that subsequently becomes infected. Treatment is primary prevention of an elevation of calcium-phosphorus product.

Metastatic calcification

Metastatic calcification occurs when calcium and phosphorus precipitate and deposit in blood vessels and tissues. This occurs when the calcium and phosphorus levels are high. High is defined by a calcium-phosphorus product of greater than 70. In order to prevent metastatic calcification it is important to decrease serum phosphorus. This is accomplished with a diet restricted for phosphorus and judicious use of phosphate binders.

Renal bone disease in pediatric patients with chronic kidney disease

Renal failure causes a metabolic acidosis. The acidosis causes displacement of calcium from the bones and retards bone growth. Hyperparathyroidism also retards bone growth. Thus, children with chronic kidney disease are of short stature. The biochemical changes along with malnutrition frequently leave children at the low end for height. Treatment of low stature includes correction of any nutritional deficiencies and chronic acidosis.

Proteinuria

Marker of kidney disease
Normal renal physiology allows for some protein to be filtered and excreted into the urine. By in large, most proteins are not filtered at the glomerulus and thus are never reabsorbed or excreted in the renal tubules. However, early marker of kidney damage is protein loss. There are different methods of urine collection but the most practical is a spot urinalysis. Spot refers to a one time, random collection of urine during the day. The urine is sent for an albumin: creatinine ratio. If the ratio exceeds 30, there is evidence of early renal disease and modification of risk factors is important.

Measurement
Urinary protein is measured to assess renal damage. The most abundant protein in the serum is albumin. Albumin is normally not filtered nor secreted in the renal tubules. However, with renal damage, albumin is filtered and excreted in the urine. One method of measuring urinary protein is

a 24-hour urine collection. The patient's urine is collected for 24 hours and is sent for albumin, creatinine and total protein. The major limitation for a 24-hour urine collection is difficulty in collecting urine over a prolonged period. Another method of measuring urinary protein is to collect a "spot" urine. The term spot refers to a random, one time collection of urine. The advantage of a spot collection is that it is a one-time void, which is easier to collect. The urine is sent for an albumin:creatinine ratio. If the ratio is >30 mg/day than urinary protein is elevated and renal disease is present. Lastly, the routine urinalysis also measures proteinuria. However, it can only detect albumin levels of greater than 300 mg/day. Thus, it is not as sensitive as the albumin:creatinine ratio which can detect albumin levels as low as 30 mg/day.

Pathophysiology of anemia of chronic kidney disease

The kidneys are important in releasing the hormone erythropoietin. Erythropoietin travels from the kidneys to the bone marrow and helps stimulate red blood cell formation. In patients with chronic kidney disease, there is nephronal loss. With less nephrons secreting adequate erythropoietin, there is less red blood cell production and hence anemia. To combat this, clinicians often give erythropoietin in patients with anemia. However, iron is also an important ingredient in red blood cell makeup. Therefore, by building iron stores in the body one can address the anemia in combination with erythropoietin if deemed necessary.

Anemia

Etiology, symptoms, and effect of dialysis
Anemia is a commonly found in uremic patients. Red blood cell production decreases in ESRD patients, and the cells that do form are frequently abnormal. Hematocrit values for a normal male are between 46 and 52%, and in a normal female, range from 40 to 45%. In the dialysis patient, the values are considerably lower with non-intervention patients leveling off in the 20-30% range. One cause of anemia in these patients is diminished erythropoietin (EPO), a hormone that stimulates the production of blood cells by bone marrow. Another is the inability to successfully absorb and use iron. In addition, the life span of the red blood cell decreases. Platelet abnormalities lead to bleeding from the gums, nose, GI tract, uterus, and skin. Symptoms of anemia include weakness, fatigue, and shortness of breath, chest pain, poor exercise tolerance, and inability to think clearly. During dialysis, the dialyzer may leak, frequent blood tests are done, and blood recovery may be incomplete. All of these are avoidable and care must be taken to reduce these causes of anemia.

Pediatric patients with chronic kidney disease
The pathophysiology of anemia in the pediatric population is similar to adults. However, the erythropoietin and iron requirements to correct the anemia are substantially higher. Erythropoietin should be administered subcutaneously. Supplemental iron needs to be administered both orally and, if needed, intravenously.

Uremia

GI complaints
Uremia is responsible for several GI complaints. Circulating uremic toxins cause nausea and vomiting in ESRD patients. The most frequent gastrointestinal complaints include the following:
- Nausea
- Poor appetite
- Metallic taste in mouth
- Vomiting

- Fetid breath (from decomposing urea)
- GI bleeding, often occult may be caused by platelet abnormalities and aggravated by the use of Heparin.
- Ammonia or hyperkalemia may cause diarrhea.
- Functional constipation and possible impactions may result from medications, diet, and lack of exercise or fluid restriction.

It is important to encourage patients to eat a high-fiber diet, exercise regularly, and if needed, use a stool softener.

Neurologic system changes
Neurologic symptoms may range from inattention to coma, depending upon the degree and cause of the uremic encephalopathy. Insomnia, restlessness, and anorexia are all seen when azotemia is present. Left unresolved, the symptoms could progress to emotional lability, lethargy, and vomiting. The most severe consequences of untreated azotemia can be coma and death. Commonly seen neurologic symptoms are anxiety, depression, agitation, and fatigue. Restless leg syndrome (RLS), in which the patient has uncontrollable urges to move the extremities when at rest, has been noted in uremia patients. Anemia and hyperphosphatemia may be contributing factors.

Metabolic disturbances
Metabolism of glucose, lipids, and protein are often found to be abnormal in uremia patients. In nondiabetic ESRD patients, the decrease of cellular sensitivity to insulin results in abnormal glucose metabolism. In type 1 diabetes, hyperglycemic and hypoglycemic swings may be severe. Dialysis may decrease the insulin requirement. In type 2 diabetics, weight reduction, increased physical activity, and the administration of hypoglycemic agents may improve their glucose metabolism. Lipoprotein metabolism and structure are altered in ESRD patients. Type 4 hyperlipoproteinemia occurs regularly in this type of patient. Low levels of carnitine, a compound that is required for the transport of fatty acids into the mitochondria, may be found to play a part in this metabolic dysfunctionProtein metabolism dysfunction may result in wasting, impaired growth, and malnutrition. Poor intake, resulting in low serum albumin, depletion of nutrients during dialysis, and abnormal metabolism are all factors that influence this process. Loss of tissue mass may be obscured by edema.

Measuring Kidney Function

GFR

The best method for measuring kidney function and tracking the progression of chronic kidney disease is through the calculation of the glomerular filtration rate (GFR). The GFR is commonly estimated by two different equations: the Cockcroft-Gault equation and the modification of diet in renal disease (MDRD) equation.

Cockcroft-Gault equation
The Cockcroft-Gault estimates the body's creatine clearance rate (CC, which itself is an estimate of GFR in mL/min) by the following:

$$CC = \frac{(140 - age) \times body\ mass}{72 \times serum\ creatinine}$$

Where *age* is in years, *body mass* is in kg, and *serum creatinine* is in mg/dL. For female patients, the result is multiplied by a factor of 0.85.

MDRD equation
The MDRD estimates the body's GFR in mL/min by the following:

$$GFR = 186 \times Serum\ Creatinine^{-1.154} \times Age^{-0.203}$$

Or alternatively:

$$GFR = 170 \times Serum\ Creatinine^{-0.999} \times Age^{-0.176} \times BUN^{-0.17} \times Albumin^{0.318}$$

Where *age* is in years, *serum creatinine* and *BUN* are in mg/dL, and *Albumin* is in g/dL. For female patients, the result is multiplied by a factor of 0.742 (or 0.762 for the second equation). For African American patients, the result is multiplied by a factor of 1.21 (or 1.18 for the second equation).

Comparing the two methods
The Cockcroft-Gault equation is easily memorized and requires only one blood test to calculate. It also adjusts for the weight of the patient. However, its accuracy is questionable since it estimates a quantity which is itelf an estimate of the quantity of interest.

The MDRD, although much more complicated, is the prefered equation because it is considered to be more accurate, particularly the alternate form of the equation. Unlike the CG, it does not account for patient weight, but it does account for ethnicity (sort of). It provides a modification only for African American patients.

The major limitation for both equations is that their accuracy falls off considerably at GFRs above 60. The equations are much more accurate for stages II – V. Both equations also rely heavily on having accurate lab results. Any significant amount of error in the lab results will render the estimates useless.

Schwartz and Counahan-Barratt equations

The Schwartz equation is used to calculate the glomerular filtration rate in children. The equation is as follows: GFR = k x 0.55 x height (cm)/Creatinine (mg/dL), where k is a constant. The Counahan-Barratt equation is: GFR = k x 0.43 x height (cm)/Creatinine (mg/dL), where k is a constant. The major difference between the two equations is the constants (k). The equations use the proportional relationship between GFR and height and creatinine. Both equations lose some accuracy as glomerular filtration rates exceed 90 mg/min/1.73m^2.

Laboratory tests needed for patients with chronic kidney disease

All patients with chronic kidney disease should be evaluated by a nephrologist. The evaluation should include the following blood work:
- Hemoglobin and hematocrit
- Iron studies
- Red blood cell indices (mean corpuscular volume and red cell distribution width)
- Electrolytes including phosphorus
- Urinalysis

The hemoglobin/hematocrit and red blood cell indices are important to evaluate those patients with anemia. Electrolyte measurements are used to adequately following the progression of CKD with estimation of glomerular filtration rates. It is also important to monitor phosphorus levels. Phosphorus is excreted by the kidney and in declining renal function, phosphorus accumulates. The urinalysis is important in evaluating proteinuria. However, the urinalysis is only effective at measuring heavy chain proteins, which are excreted at greater than 300 mg/dl. If less than 300 mg/dl of protein is excreted one can perform either a 24-hour urine collection for protein or a spot urine microalbumin/creatinine ratio. Less common tests ordered include erythropoietin levels and parathyroid hormone levels.

Imaging modalities to detect underlying causes of chronic kidney disease

The most common imaging modality used is the ultrasound. Renal ultrasounds reveal shape, size and contour of the kidneys. It can help identify hydronephrosis, cysts and tumors. Also, commonly used are CAT scans with/without intravenous contrast. Radiocontrast must be used with caution in patients with chronic kidney disease for it has been well documented to be nephrotoxic. However, cat scans provide a more precise image of the kidneys. Less commonly used imaging includes intravenous pyelograms, nuclear scans and MRI.

Decreased GFR without kidney damage

Decreased glomerular filtration rate without kidney damaged is defined as a GFR between 60-89 mL/min/1.73m^2 without obvious signs of kidney failure. This is usually attributed to the aging process but can also be seen in young adults and children. The prognosis of decreased GFR is good and progression to stage V CKD is unlikely. Moreover, these patients may not present the sequale of chronic kidney disease including anemia and bone disease.

Preferred method of renal replacement in pediatric patients

Nearly all pediatric patients with renal disease should be placed on the transplant list. While awaiting transplant the preferred method of renal replacement is peritoneal dialysis. Peritoneal dialysis affords the child freedom to attend school and live a more normal life. Hemodialysis is reserved for those patients when peritoneal dialysis is contraindicated or does not have the support structure.

Use of dialyzers and hemodialysis machines in pediatric patients

The special use of dialyzers in children is aimed at the smaller body surface area. Hollow fiber dialyzers are the preferred dialyzer because of low compliance. The dialyzer surface area is also smaller to accommodate the smaller surface area. Dialyzer reuse is seldom used in pediatrics.

Hemodialysis machines, however, do not differ from adult machines. Adult machines can be calibrated to adjust to pediatric volumes.

Complications

Aluminum in patients with chronic kidney disease

Major sources of aluminum
Previously, aluminum-based phosphate binders were commonly used and were a major source of aluminum toxicity. Aluminum helped bind phosphate in the gut. However, aluminum would also be absorbed and deposited into bones and cause dementia. Today, while aluminum-based phosphate binders are not readily used, other medicines may contain aluminum. These include the commonly used antacid aluminum hydroxide (trade name Maalox). Caution must be taken in using aluminum hydroxide in patients with chronic kidney disease. Overuse of antacids containing aluminum will lead to toxicity. Another source of aluminum is through the water system used for dialysis. Today, water purification systems have improved and water-testing methods are more sensitive today, preventing some causes of aluminum toxicity.

Toxicity
Aluminum is excreted by the kidneys. In patients with renal disease, the ability to excrete aluminum is hindered. Aluminum toxicity was a much larger problem when aluminum based phosphate binders were used. The aluminum would be absorbed by the gut and accumulate over time. Treatment of acute aluminum toxicity is via hemodialysis with a low aluminum dialysate concentration. Osteomalacia, dementia, anemia and hypercalcemia are products of chronic exposure to aluminum. Prevention of aluminum exposure is hugely important with avoidance of aluminum based phosphate binders and frequent monitoring of dialysis water system for elevated aluminum levels.

Complications: The major complications of aluminum toxicity include:
- Acute aluminum toxicity
- Dementia
- Hypercalcemia (by displacing calcium in bony matrix)
- Anemia
- Osteomalacia

Acute aluminum toxicity presents as an acute change in mental status. Patients need urgent and daily hemodialysis with low aluminum in the dialysate solution to remove the excess aluminum. Dementia is caused by chronic exposure to aluminum. The most common source of chronic aluminum exposure is a contaminated water system with high levels of aluminum. Chronic exposure to aluminum will also lead to osteomalacia (aluminum depositing in bone) and hypercalcemia (aluminum replacing calcium in bone).

Interventions

Aims of treatment of chronic kidney disease

All patients with chronic kidney disease should have the following goals of treatment:
- Identify and treat comorbid conditions
- Diagnosis specific therapy
- Slowing the progression of chronic kidney disease
- Identifying and modifying cardiovascular risk factors
- Preparation for renal replacement therapy
- Renal replacement therapy if clinically indicated

Management necessary in treating each stage of chronic kidney disease

The management necessary in the treatment of each stage of chronic kidney disease is explained below:
- Stage I (GFR >90)—Diagnose and treat comorbid conditions, eliminate and/or treat known risk factors for chronic renal disease, slow the progression of cardiovascular disease, possible use of ace inhibitors or angiotensin receptor blockers.
- Stage II (GFR 60-89)—Estimate the progression of renal disease, eliminate and/or treat known risk factors for chronic renal disease, use ace inhibitors or angiotensin receptor blockers.
- Stage III (GFR 30-59)—Evaluate and treat complications of renal disease, use ace inhibitors or angiotensin receptor blockers,
- Stage IV (GFR 15-29)—Prepare for renal replacement therapy, use ace inhibitors or angiotensin receptor blockers if tolerated.
- Stage V (GFR <15)—Renal replacement via hemodialysis or peritoneal dialysis or transplant if uremia present.

Interventions shown to increase rate of decline of renal disease

The following is a list of interventions which are currently recommend by the Kidney Disease Outcomes Quality Initiative (KDOQI):
- Strict glycemic control
- Blood pressure control to optimal levels
- Use of ace inhibitors or angiotensin receptor blockers
- Correction of anemia
- Management of hyperlipidemia
- Dietary protein restriction

All of the stated interventions help control the rate of decline of GFR and slows the progression towards end stage renal disease.

Initial assessment of CKD patient

Initial assessment of the CKD patient should include the following:
- Comprehensive personal and familial history
- Complete physical examination
- Complete blood count
- Blood chemistry
- Complete urinalysis
- Renal ultrasound

Goals of comprehensive assessment
The goals of the comprehensive assessment are as follows:
- Distinguish between acute and chronic kidney disease
- Establish the etiology of the disease
- Determine the GFR
- Evaluate the rate of progression
- Analyze cardiovascular risk
- Assess protein excretion
- Gauge reversible damage
- Determine life style risks
- Evaluate dialysis vs. transplant
- Assess medications
- Determine complications of primary disease

Final diagnosis of CKD during initial assessment of patient with kidney disease

The factors that influence the final diagnosis of CKD include the size of the kidney (determined by renal ultrasound), hemoglobin level, and ongoing assessment of renal function. In acute kidney disease, size is not a factor while in chronic disease, the evidence of small renal size in addition to the reduction of GFR for more than 3 months are indicative of chronic kidney disease. Assessing reversible renal dysfunction is an important step in determining chronic disease. Evaluation of extracellular fluid volume (ECFV), hypotension or extreme hypertension, cardiac failure, urinary obstruction, sepsis, and nephrotoxins is helpful in determining if damage could be reversible.

Optimal blood pressures for patients with and without proteinuria

According to the Joint National Committee for the prevention, detection, evaluation, and treatment of high blood pressure (JNC VI), the optimal blood pressure is a systolic of <120 and diastolic of <80. This is particularly relevant for those patients with proteinuria. Lowering blood pressure has been shown to dramatically reduce proteinuria and slow the progression of chronic kidney disease. However, in patients without documented proteinuria or risk factors for chronic kidney disease, acceptable blood pressures are systolic of <130 and diastolic of <85. The take home message is lower is better.

Importance of managing hypertension

Hypertension can either cause or be a consequence of chronic kidney disease. It is a major public health risk and optimal management is important. Uncontrolled blood pressure can lead to coronary artery disease, stroke, kidney failure, left ventricular hypertrophy and congestive heart failure. The current guidelines advise that ace inhibitors be the agent of choice in managing hypertension. Multiple studies have found a decrease in all cause mortality and morbidity in patients on ace inhibitors. Angiotensin receptor blockers are also acceptable alternatives to ace inhibitors.

Importance of blood pressure management in patients with diabetes

Diabetes places patients at high risk for renal failure. Poor glycemic control causes renal damage and proteinuria. Up to 40% of patients with diabetes will progress to end stage renal disease and require dialysis. The concomitant presence of hypertension only exacerbates the risk and progression of chronic kidney disease. Therefore, it is imperative that patients with diabetes receive special attention in controlling both the serum glucose but also blood pressure. According to the Joint National committee for the prevention, detection, evaluation, and treatment of high blood pressure (JNC VI), the optimal blood pressure is 120/80. All diabetics should receive pharmacotherapy as well as diet and exercise regimens to achieve the stated goal. Again, the best agents in controlling blood pressure and reducing proteinuria are ace inhibitors. Angiotensin receptor blockers are excellent alternatives to ace inhibitors.

Pre-dialysis assessment

Pre-dialysis assessment is a very important step in preparing the patient for maintenance dialysis. Pre-dialysis assessments should include the following in order to best prepare a patient for maintenance dialysis:
- Afford suitable group and individualized predialysis education
- Assess social and psychological needs
- Determine home dialysis vs. hospital based treatment
- Decide on peritoneal dialysis vs. hemodialysis
- Rectify reversible factors precluding preferred dialysis mode
- Evaluate and treat infections (HIV, methicillin-resistant Staphylococcus aureus-MRSA, vancomycin-resistant Enterococcus-VRE, hepatitis B and C)
- Create dialysis access to permit optimal time for initiation
- Attain consent for ANZDATA (Australia and New Zealand Dialysis and Transplant Registry) compilation

Therapies in addition to dialysis

Dialysis alone cannot fully replace the function of a normal kidney. Supplemental therapies are extremely important in assuring the success of dialysis, these include the following:
- Suitable water and sodium intake for regulation of extracellular fluid volume (ECFV) and plasma osmolality
- Dietary restriction or supplementation for potassium balance
- Phosphate binders (Calcitriol) when indicated for calcium/phosphate balance
- $NaHCO_3$ for acid-base balance
- Avoidance of excess magnesium to maintain magnesium levels
- Calcitriol as needed for activation of 25-hydroxy cholecalciferol
- Angiotensin converting enzyme inhibitor (ACEI) or angiotensin receptor blocker (ARB) for synthesis of renin-angiotensin
- Erythropoietin, or similar, for synthesis of erythropoietin

Tracking glomerular filtration rates

The rate of decline of kidney function increases in patients with chronic kidney disease. As the glomerular filtration rate decreases, the rate of decline towards dialysis also increases. Tracking the glomerular filtration rate aids clinicians in assessing how quickly renal function is declining. It also helps in assessing the effects of interventions on declining renal functions. Furthermore, as patients progress from stage to stage in chronic kidney disease, clinical interventions and management also change. For example, if a patient progresses from stage III to stage IV CKD, preparation must be made for renal replacement therapy. This includes both gaining access as well as preparing the patient and social support network for the emotional impact of dialysis.

Importance of treating chronic kidney disease as it relates to the cardiovascular system

The leading cause of death in patients with renal failure is not renal related complications but rather coronary artery disease. Large epidemiological trials have clearly demonstrated that chronic kidney disease is an independent risk factor for coronary artery disease and cardiovascular related deaths. Renal failure is frequently associated with diabetes and hypertension (both known risk factors for cardiac disease). Glycemic control and treatment of high blood pressure are important risk modifiers of renal disease and cardiovascular deaths. Patients with chronic kidney disease should decrease salt intake, exercise and stop smoking. Furthermore, any elevations of cholesterol should be treated with diet, exercise and medications if necessary. Finally, ace inhibitors have been shown to be efficacious in slowing the progression of chronic kidney disease and in treating patients with heart failure. Ace inhibitors are also important in controlling blood pressure and have been shown to decrease cholesterol levels to some extent.

Evaluating bone metabolism

All patients with chronic kidney disease need the following blood tests in evaluating renal bone disease:
- Serum calcium
- Serum phosphorus
- Parathyroid hormone

The serum calcium is necessary to ensure that calcium levels are not dangerously low. Serum phosphorus is important to ensure that phosphorus levels are not high. Moreover, the product of serum calcium and phosphorus is important in determining a patient's risk for metastatic calcification. The calcium-phosphorus product should be kept below 70. Finally, the serum parathyroid hormone needs to be checked. In patients with chronic kidney disease, the PTH should be kept at about 1.5 – 2 times the upper limits of normal. Low PTH levels places patients at risk for adynamic bone disease. High PTH levels places patients at risk for osteoporosis and fractures.

Recommendations on dietary phosphorus restriction

Most dietary phosphorus comes in the form of protein. Therefore, dietary protein restriction would greatly aid in lowering phosphorus intake. However, this only applies to patients with chronic kidney disease (CKD) Stages II-IV. In patients with stage V CKD, protein restriction is known to cause malnutrition. In fact, patients on dialysis frequently need more protein to ensure adequate nutrition. Thus, in patients with CKD Stages II-IV, protein restriction aids in lowering phosphorus. However, in patients with CKD Stage V, protein restriction is harmful. Therefore, CKD Stage V patients will require phosphate binders and elimination of dietary phosphorus from non-protein sources.

Limitations of dietary calcium intake in patients with elevated phosphorus levels

The limits of total daily calcium intake should not exceed 2000 mg. Furthermore, only 1500 mg of elemental calcium is permitted daily when given a calcium based phosphate binder. The rationale of limiting calcium intake is that excess calcium intake will result in increased calcium absorption. If too much calcium is absorbed, the calcium-phosphorus product may exceed the set limits of 70. A calcium-phosphorus product of greater than 70 leaves the patient susceptible to metastatic calcification and the more rare condition of calciphylaxis.

Anemia of chronic kidney disease

Benefits of treatment
Treating anemia of chronic kidney disease has both a survival and quality of life benefit.
- In patients on hemodialysis, treating anemia has led to overall survival. The mortality rates decreased overall in patients treated to appropriate hemoglobin levels.
- Other benefits include a reduction in left ventricular hypertrophy and decreased rates of hospitalizations.
- Moreover, the quality of life for patients improves. The exercise capacity is improved as measured by standardized six-minute walk tests.
- Overall, both survival and quality of life improved greatly with appropriate treatment of anemia.
- Conversely, not treating or under-treating anemia leads to increased mortality and decreased quality of life.

Acceptable hemoglobin levels
According to the current National Kidney Foundation's Kidney Disease Outcomes Quality Initiative (KDOQI), acceptable hemoglobin levels for men and postmenopausal women is >12 and premenopausal women is >11. Why the disparity? The reasons are two fold:
- Men have more body mass and thus will require more hemoglobin
- Premenopausal women are still actively menstruating. The monthly blood loss will result in lower hemoglobin levels. This combined with low body masses allows for premenopausal women to have lower hemoglobin levels. Furthermore, postmenopausal women are no longer menstruating. Thus, they are held to the higher standard of >12. A hemoglobin level of under 12 would indicate a possibility of occult blood loss, namely colon cancer.

Workup
Anemia of chronic kidney disease is indicated in men and postmenopausal women with hemoglobin levels <12 and premenopausal women with hemoglobin levels <11. The workup should consist of the following blood test:
- Hemoglobin/hematocrit
- Red blood cell indices
- Iron studies
- Tsats (iron/total iron binding capacity x 100)
- Reticulocyte counts
- Occult fecal blood

A less common test includes serum erythropoietin. Low levels of erythropoietin in the absence of other causes of anemia suggest that failing kidneys are the cause of the anemia and appropriate supplementation is required.

Goals of therapy
The most basic goal is to achieve a hemoglobin level > 12 in men and postmenopausal women and > 11 in premenopausal women. However, achieving that goal is more complicated. Foremost, the body must have adequate iron stores. A lack of iron will lead to iron deficiency anemia and any further medicines, including erythropoietin will not be effective. Therefore, iron studies must be drawn. Ferritin levels (a measure of active iron) must be greater than 100. Another marker for iron stores is the iron/total iron binding capacity saturation percentage or Tsats. The appropriate Tsat level should exceed 20%. Anything less than 20% and iron must be replaced. Finally, erythropoietin levels should be drawn. If the level is low (often it is in patients with chronic kidney disease) than erythropoietin should be given to help correct the anemia. Remember, without the iron, erythropoietin is ineffective for it will stimulate red blood cells without the very important iron component needed.

Drawing ferritin and Tsats
Ferritin is an indication of the amount of active iron stores in the body. Tsats stand for transferrin saturation percentage. It is derived by the following ratio: iron/total iron binding capacity multiplied by 100 to give a percentage. In formula form it is more commonly written as: Fe/TIBC x 100.

The Tsats are another indicator for iron stores in the body. Both the ferritin and Tsats will indicate if total body iron stores are low. If these markers for total body iron are indeed low, than one can assume the anemia is secondary to iron deficiency. Supplemental iron must be given. Furthermore, trending the ferritin and Tsats will aid the clinician in tracking response to therapy. The current guidelines stipulate that the ferritin should be >100 and Tsats >20%.

Drawing hemoglobin/hematocrit
The hemoglobin/hematocrit is the mainstay of documenting the presence of anemia and is necessary to follow progression of therapy. In order to diagnose anemia, the hemoglobin and hematocrit levels must be below the accepted lower limits of normal (<12 in men and postmenopausal women and <11 in premenopausal women). If the hemoglobin/hematocrit is below normal, than a work up of the type of anemia is necessary. It is important for clinicians to recognize that the anemia present is indeed secondary to chronic kidney disease and not another mechanism. Finally, trending hemoglobin/hematocrit levels is necessary to ensure appropriate responses to therapy.

Drawing reticulocyte counts
Reticulocytes are the precursors to mature red blood cells. They are released by the bone marrow and are indication of anemia if their levels are high. The physiological response to low hemoglobin/hematocrit is to stimulate the release of erythropoietin from the kidneys. Erythropoietin acts on the bone marrow to increase red cell production. The increase in red blood cell demand will cause an increase in reticulocyte production. If, however, the bone marrow is not functioning properly, the reticulocyte count will not respond appropriately to erythropoietin. Thus, in the presence of an anemia (low hemoglobin/hematocrit), a low reticulocyte count will indicate a bone marrow problem. In this instance a further workup is needed and supplemental iron and erythropoietin will not be effective.

Drawing red blood cell indices

The most important red blood cell index is the MCV or mean corpuscular volume. It is an indicator of how much hemoglobin and iron are within each red blood cell. If the hemoglobin and iron levels are low, the MCV will be low. However, excess hemoglobin or iron does not indicate a high MCV. A high MCV is usually found in patients with vitamin B12 and folate deficiencies. The other indices are also indicators of low iron or vitamin B12 and folate. This is just another measure to help clinicians narrow down the cause of the anemia. Again, a low MCV leads towards a diagnosis of iron deficiency anemia.

Examining fecal occult blood

A frequent cause of anemia is the loss of blood via the gastrointestinal tract. Common causes of gastrointestinal blood loss include:
- Colon cancer
- Peptic and gastric ulcers
- Diverticulosis

The loss of blood will cause an anemia. In order to diagnose blood loss from the gastrointestinal tract, fecal hemoccult cards are used. The cards help identify blood loss which is not readily detectable with the naked eye. Blood loss via this route will help clinicians identify that the anemia is not necessarily due to chronic kidney disease and a further workup is need.

Upper limits of acceptable ranges for treatment

In men and postmenopausal women, the target hemoglobin is >12. In premenopausal women, the target hemoglobin is >11. However, iron supplementation can lead to adverse effects, chiefly cardiac, lung and liver dysfunction. In order to monitor iron therapy, the ferritin and Tsats are followed. Iron supplementation should be stopped if the ferritin exceeds 800 and the Tsat exceeds 50%. Again, higher levels than those stated are associated with iron overload states and can lead to cardiac, lung and liver dysfunction.

Administering iron

Iron is almost universally replenished orally. In fact, that is the preferred method. However, iron has some side effects, most notably constipation. Some patients may not be able to absorb iron because of gastrointestinal diseases including some malabsorption syndromes. Additionally, some patients do not adequately respond to oral iron therapy. Intravenous iron is the solution for those patients who cannot absorb iron or do not respond appropriately. Intravenous iron is administered during dialysis sessions with dosing according to their ferritin and Tsat levels.

Patient education about stages of ESRD

The chronic kidney disease patient should be educated about the stages of ESRD. Some of the benefits of pre-ESRD education are as follows:
- Decreases stress for patient and family members
- Improves the mortality and morbidity rates
- Increases self-care, aids in decision making
- Improves the ability to maintain employment
- Allows for informed decision making when replacement therapy is indicated

The American Association of Kidney Patients (AAKP) has created numerous programs to help those living with chronic kidney disease. Kidney Options is one such program that is co-sponsored by

AAKP and Fresenius Medical Care North America. Informational materials are available on their website, through a newsletter, in brochures, and at local patient education venues. AAKP also works with Baxter Healthcare and the Stay in Touch program and provides educational mailings customized to the current needs of the patient as well as a toll-free hotline and a website.

Diet
The registered dietitian plays an important role in educating the ESRD patient. A proper diet may be beneficial by producing the following results:
- Delaying the need for dialysis
- Reducing the complications (phosphorus restriction to prevent bone complications)
- Providing adequate nutrition (improve morbidity and mortality)
- Improving the quality of life by customizing the diet (ethnic, lifestyle, variables)

Protein restriction, when implemented in concert with proper caloric intake, can be helpful in controlling uremic symptoms and in reducing the nitrogenous wastes. Kidney Disease Outcomes Quality Initiative (K/DOQI) recommends that patients with a GFR of less than $60mL/1.73m^2$ should have their nutritional status, protein, and caloric intake assessed. When teaching the ESRD patient about proper diet, protein requirements play an important role. Areas that should be covered include the amount of protein that needs to be included in the daily intake. The latest research suggests $1.2 \pm 0.2g/kg/day$ of protein with the higher range reserved for protein-malnourished patients. Half of the daily protein should come from high-biologic value protein (animal protein). The other half may be derived from certain fruits, vegetables, and grains. One cup of corn, potato, peas, pasta, or rice (cooked) contains approximately 4 grams of protein.

Review of medications

Every chronic kidney disease patient should have all medicines reviewed at each visit. According to the National Kidney Foundation, the following parameters should be reviewed:
- Dose adjustment based on glomerular filtration rate
- Detection of drug interactions
- Therapeutic drug monitoring
- Detection of adverse drug reactions on renal function

Treating conditions commonly found in ESRD patient

Although there are no medications currently available to reverse or cure kidney failure, several drugs have proven valuable in treating conditions commonly found in the ESRD patient. Drugs administered in CKD patients include the following:
- Cinacalcet HCl (Senispar) is a drug used for lowering the level of parathyroid hormone (PTH) in the blood. CKD interferes with metabolism of calcium, phosphate, and vitamin D. CKD leads to a condition known as hyperparathyroidism in which elevated levels of PTH if left untreated may lead to uremic bone disease. This is an oral medication. Possible side effects associated with Senispar are nausea, vomiting, and transient low blood calcium levels.
- Furosemide (Lasix) and bumetanide (Bumex) are commonly used diuretics. They are available in oral form and as injections. Side effects may include dizziness, dry mouth, frequent urination, and weakness.

Over the counter medications for ESRD patients

Over the counter medications may be ordered for the ESRD patient. Over-the-counter medications that may be prescribed for the ESRD patient include the following:
- Sodium Bicarbonate is often used for treatment of metabolic acidosis, a condition that occurs due to the damaged kidney's inability to synthesize ammonia and excrete hydrogen ions. It is administered orally when taken as an over-the-counter medication. Sodium levels must be monitored when this medication is taken.
- Calcium Carbonate and Calcium Acetate are oral medications that are used to bind phosphate for preventing bone loss due to abnormally high phosphate levels in the blood. Side effects may include constipation, slow heart rate, and loss of appetite.

Hypertension

According to the Seventh Report of the Joint National Committee on Prevention, Detection, Evaluation, and Treatment of High Blood Pressure (JNC 7), hypertension is divided in to the following stages:

Stage	Blood Pressure Range
Normal	<120/<80 mmHg
Prehypertension	120-139/80-89 mmHg
Stage 1	140-159/90-99 mmHg
Stage 2	>160/>100 mmHg

Antihypertensive medications

The most common medications include:
- Thiazide diuretics—Block sodium and chloride at the distal convoluted tubule resulting in excess water excretion
- Beta blockers—Act on B1 receptors on the heart to slow heart rate and thus, cardiac output
- Ace-Inhibitors—Act by blocking angiotensin converting enzyme which is crucial to the conversion of angiotensin I to angiotensin II (potent vasoconstrictor)
- Angiotensin Receptor Blockers—Block the angiotensin II receptors
- Calcium channel blockers—Slow the heart rate as well as vasodilate the peripheral circulation

Treatment of hyperparathyroidism

Two medications prescribed for the treatment of hyperparathyroidism are as follows:
- Paricalcitol (Zemplar) injection is an aggressive treatment for secondary hyperparathyroidism. The usual administration route for paricalcitol (Zemplar) is intravenous. This medication decreases the PTH levels and has a negligible effect on phosphorus and calcium. Digitalis toxicity must be monitored if hypercalcemia is present. Paricalcitol is contraindicated in patients with vitamin D toxicity and hypercalcemia.
- Doxercalciferol (Hectorol) is also used to control PTH and hyperparathyroidism. It may be administered intravenously or orally. The patient needs to be monitored for hypercalcemia, hyperphosphatemia, and hypoparathyroidism while on Hectorol.

Ace inhibitors

Chronic kidney disease is frequently accompanied by protein loss in the urine. The inability of the kidneys to retain protein is not only an indication of renal failure but is injurious to the nephron. Proteins are harmful to the kidney and measures to slow protein filtration and loss is important to prevent kidney disease progression. Ace inhibitors act by decreasing the amount of protein loss in the kidney. They do so by blocking the actions of the angiotensin-converting enzyme. This enzyme helps release angiotensin II, which is a potent vasoconstrictor. By blocking this enzyme, the renal arteries (particularly the efferent arteriole) are allowed to vasodilate. The vasodilatory effects of ace inhibitors slow the amount of protein being delivered and filtered at the kidneys. Thus, protein loss is curbed and progression of chronic kidney disease delayed.

Phosphate binders

There are three main categories of phosphate binders:
- Aluminum based
- Calcium based
- Non-calcium based

Aluminum based phosphate binders were used to bind phosphate in the gut and prevent its absorption. However, significant side effects of aluminum including osteomalacia and dementia have eliminated aluminum as a viable option. Calcium based phosphate binders are the most commonly used. They bind phosphorus in the gut with some absorption of elemental calcium. The main side effect of calcium based binders is hypercalcemia. Finally, non-calcium based binders are new to the market and are increasingly popular. They are polymers that bind to intestinal phosphorus and have few side effects in contrast to aluminum and calcium based binders.

Phosphorus levels should be kept at normal to high normal levels in patients with chronic kidney disease. Dietary restriction should be the first attempt at reducing phosphorus levels. However, in patients with persistently elevated phosphorus despite dietary restriction, phosphate binders should be used. In patients with chronic kidney disease stages III – IV, calcium based binders are the first choice. Calcium based binders are preferred in this patient population for the supplemental calcium will aid in preserving bone integrity and reducing PTH levels. However, in patients with stage V CKD, either calcium based or non-calcium based binders are preferred. The difference is that in patients with stage V CKD, they often have higher phosphorus levels. Any supplemental calcium absorbed with calcium based binders may precipitate metastatic calcification. Therefore, non-calcium based binders are equally as effective in patients with stage V CKD.

Management of hypercalcemia in patients with chronic kidney disease stage V

In patients on renal replacement therapy and with a serum calcium level above 10.2 the following measures should be taken to reduce serum calcium. First, in patients taking calcium based phosphate binders the dose should be reduced. If that does not work, the alternative of using a non-calcium based binder should be implemented. Second, in patients taking supplemental vitamin D the dose should be reduced or eliminated. Finally, if the aforementioned steps did not adequately reduce serum calcium levels than using a lower calcium dialysate solution should be used. Hopefully, dialysate solutions with lower calcium levels will help eliminate excess serum calcium with each dialysis session.

Vitamin D supplementation

Patients with chronic kidney disease are subject to hyperparathyroidism. In order to maintain parathyroid hormone levels at acceptable levels, the serum calcium and phosphorus must be at near normal levels. Moreover, a deficiency of vitamin D will lead to excess release of PTH. Thus, in patients with PTH levels above acceptable limits as determined by the stage of chronic kidney disease a vitamin D level must be checked. If the vitamin D level is below normal, supplemental vitamin D should be offered. Hopefully, the vitamin D will lower PTH levels to acceptable levels (1.5 – 2 times normal). Serial vitamin D and PTH levels along with serum calcium and phosphorus need to be checked to monitor therapy.

Limitations in patients with chronic kidney disease
Patients with chronic kidney disease and elevated PTH levels with concomitant low vitamin D stores will need vitamin D supplementation. Vitamin D is administered in oral form and it will increase absorption of calcium and phosphorus. Yet, caution must be taken so as not to raise the serum calcium and phosphorus levels to above acceptable limits. If the serum calcium becomes elevated, a lower dosage or discontinuation of vitamin D is indicated. If the serum phosphorus becomes elevated, addition of a phosphate binder or discontinuation of vitamin D is indicated.

Hypocalcemia

In patients with low serum calcium levels care must be taken to ensure that the patient is not symptomatic. Signs of low calcium include tetany, bronchospasm, muscle twitching, and most severely seizures. Supplemental calcium should come in the form of oral calcium salts and vitamin D. Again, caution must be taken in supplementing calcium. Overzealous calcium supplementation could result in hypercalcemia and precipitate calcium deposition in tissues and vessels.

Erythropoietin

Side effects
The most common side effects of erythropoietin include the following:
- Hypertension
- Seizures
- Increased clotting and hyperkalemia

As erythropoietin takes effect some patients will see an elevation of their blood pressure. Proper monitoring and increasing antihypertensive medicines may be necessary in some patients. While increases in seizure activity, clotting and hyperkalemia have been reported, there is no need to more closely monitor patients for these side effects. Furthermore, there are no recommended prophylactic measures necessary to prevent the onset of seizures or clotting. There is no role for antiepileptic or anticoagulation prophylactically in patients on erythropoietin.

Monitoring of hemoglobin levels
According to the national kidney foundation, the hemoglobin and hematocrit levels should be monitored every 1 to 2 weeks following the initiation of erythropoietin. The erythropoietin dose should be given until a stable hemoglobin level is reached. If the hemoglobin is below the stated goals of >12 in men and postmenopausal women and >11 in premenopausal women, than a higher dose of erythropoietin should be given. The cycle of dose adjustments and monitoring should be continued until the target is achieved. Once the target is achieved, hemoglobin can be monitored every 2-4 weeks.

Delivering erythropoietin
Erythropoietin is most effective when administered via the subcutaneous route. It can also be given intravenously. While most studies of erythropoietin have been through the intravenous route, subcutaneous is the preferred method. Foremost, it achieves higher levels of hemoglobin than the intravenous route, is less expensive and less dosing is required. The one major drawback to subcutaneous administration is the discomfort to the patient and the frequent changing of skin sites with each dose. Erythropoietin is administered based on dry weight and can be given with each dialysis session or once monthly depending on the manufacturer.

Alternatives to subcutaneous injections: If a patient does not tolerate subcutaneous administration of erythropoietin, the alternative would be intravenous. Intravenous erythropoietin is less effective in raising the hemoglobin/hematocrit level and is more expensive. However, it is the best alternate to subcutaneous injections. The dose of intravenous erythropoietin should be increased by 50% as compared to subcutaneous dosing. In hemodialysis patients, the intravenous form should be given through either the arterial or venous port. The intravenous forms are given once per week in contrast to the three times per week subcutaneous method.

Maintaining patient compliance with subcutaneous erythropoietin injections
The best method of maintaining patient compliance is through patient education. It is important for all patients to understand the importance of treating anemia, but also to take erythropoietin subcutaneously. The subcutaneous delivery to erythropoietin has been shown to increase the hemoglobin/hematocrit response more effectively and is less expensive. Another method for increasing compliance is to rotate injection sites so as to minimize local irritation. One should also use the smallest possible gauge needle (usually 29). Moreover, using a multi-dose preparation containing benzyl alcohol will help compliance. Benzyl alcohol acts as a local anesthetic, which helps minimize any pain. Finally, encourage the patients to self-administer the injections. This will help empower the patient and allow them to take control over their therapy.

Limitations of giving erythropoietin intravenously
Intravenous erythropoietin should be avoided for the following reasons:
- It is less effective than subcutaneous regimens in raising the hemoglobin/hematocrit level.
- It is more expensive.
- It requires intravenous access.

Studies have clearly demonstrated that the subcutaneous route of erythropoietin is more effective in treating anemia than the intravenous method. Furthermore, intravenous erythropoietin is far more expensive and will pose deterrence to both dialysis facilities and patients. Finally, in patients on peritoneal dialysis and those with chronic kidney disease stages II – IV, the need to obtain intravenous access is very cumbersome. Most patients will not want a needle stick every week to receive their erythropoietin dose. In hemodialysis patients, the erythropoietin can be given via either the arterial or venous lines at any point during the session.

Erythropoietin treatment failure

The most common cause of erythropoietin treatment failure is iron deficiency. Adequate iron stores are necessary to ensure erythropoietin's efficacy. Less common causes include:
- Infection and inflammation
- Chronic blood loss
- Osteitis fibrosa
- Aluminum toxicity
- Hemoglobinopathies
- Folate or vitamin B12 deficiency
- Multiple myeloma
- Malnutrition
- Hemolysis

The underlying conditions should be treated to ensure adequate responses to erythropoietin. In cases where erythropoietin therapy is refractory, patients with anemia should be transfused with packed red blood cells.

Chronic blood loss: Chronic blood loss always leads to iron deficiency. Any mechanism that causes iron deficiency will lead to erythropoietin treatment failure. The most common causes of chronic blood loss include:
- Gastrointestinal blood loss
- Menstruation
- Frequent blood draws in hemodialysis patients

Gastrointestinal blood loss is usually due to:
- Colorectal cancer
- Diverticulosis
- Peptic and gastric ulcers

Premenopausal women are always at increased risk for iron deficiency anemia because of menstruation. Hemodialysis patients frequently have their blood taken before and after each dialysis session. The chronic phlebotomy leads to iron losses and depletion of total body iron stores. All patients with chronic blood loss will frequently need iron supplementation.

Infection/inflammation: Chronic infections and inflammatory states have been well documented as causes of erythropoietin treatment failure. The most common causes of infections include:
- Vascular access site infections
- Chronic osteomyelitis
- Human immunodeficiency virus

The most common chronic inflammatory states include surgical patients and patients with chronic rheumatological conditions. Treatment of the underlying condition is instrumental in resolving erythropoietin treatment failure. The mechanism of infectious/inflammatory states as causing erythropoietin failure is poorly understood.

Aluminum toxicity: Aluminum toxicity occurs when patients with chronic kidney disease take certain phosphate binders. Older phosphate binders used to contain aluminum, which helped bind phosphorus in the gastrointestinal tract and limit its absorption. The use of aluminum can build in patients and deposit in bone. Bony deposition of aluminum can lead to bone marrow failure and thus resistance to erythropoietin.

Osteitis fibrosa: Osteitis fibrosa is found in many patients with chronic kidney disease. In response to phosphorus retention, parathyroid hormone levels increase. Parathyroid hormone functions to lower serum phosphorus while concomitantly increasing serum calcium. The major body store for calcium is bone. The increase in parathyroid hormone causes increased bone turnover. The increase in bone turnover also affects the makeup of bone marrow (the place where red blood cell production takes place). Increased bone activity leads to fibrosis of the bone marrow. With fibrosis of the bone marrow, there is no room for erythropoietin's ability to stimulate red blood cell production.

Folate or vitamin B12 deficiency
Folate and vitamin B12 are also essential for proper hemoglobin synthesis. A deficiency in either one will result in a macrocytic anemia. Anemia caused by folate or b12 deficiency must be corrected. While there is no direct correlation between folate and b12 and erythropoietin's mechanism of action, a macrocytic anemia must first be corrected prior to seeing any response to erythropoietin. Erythropoietin increases red blood cell production, but will not be effective if vital elements (folate and b12) for hemoglobin synthesis are missing.

Hemoglobinopathies: The most common hemoglobinopathy encountered is sickle cell disease. Sickle cell disease is a condition where hemoglobin does not function normally. This leads to a loss of oxygen carrying capacity. Erythropoietin will increase bone marrow production of defective red blood cells. The red blood cells produced will not transport oxygen effectively, rendering erythropoietin relatively ineffective. Other less common causes of hemoglobinopathies include alpha and beta thalassemia, most commonly found in persons of Asian descent.

Malnutrition: Many patients with chronic kidney disease, particularly patients on hemodialysis are frequently malnourished. Malnutrition is associated with the loss of essential and nonessential vitamins and minerals. The lack of nutrition will presumably not provide the required elements in hemoglobin and red blood cell production. This will, of course, render erythropoietin ineffective. The bone marrow will not respond appropriately if the essential requirements for red blood cell synthesis are not present.

Hemolysis: Hemolysis is frequently found when dialysate solutions are contaminated and kinks in the lines are found. Hemolysis causes acute red blood cell destruction. Erythropoietin will stimulate the bone marrow to produce red blood cells. Yet, newly formed red blood cells are destroyed, and will serve no purpose. It is important that the cause of the hemolysis is found and treated prior to initiating treatment with erythropoietin.

Administering iron along with erythropoietin
Erythropoietin stimulates the bone marrow to produce red blood cells. Red blood cells are largely made of hemoglobin, the protein necessary for oxygen transport. The main component of hemoglobin is iron. Iron is instrumental in hemoglobin's ability to carry oxygen from the lungs to the tissues. If erythropoietin stimulates red blood cell production, the body must be prepared to accommodate the increase in demand. The most important body store in this instance will be iron. If the body is does not have adequate iron stores, erythropoietin will essentially be ineffective. This is because erythropoietin will stimulate red blood cells without their most important ingredient: iron.

Erythropoietin therapy without iron supplementation
As long as anemia persists, erythropoietin is indicated. Furthermore, erythropoietin is indicated as maintenance therapy to maintain appropriate hemoglobin levels. But iron is only indicated if iron stores are below normal. Iron supplementation should continue until body stores are completely replenished. Caution must be taken with iron supplementation so as not to cause an iron overload state. Finally, hemodialysis patients frequently provide blood samples before and after each dialysis session. This phlebotomy leaves them in a chronic iron deficiency state. Therefore, it is frequently common to find hemodialysis patients taking both erythropoietin and iron as maintenance therapy.

Health care team members

The following are members of the health care team who support patients with chronic kidney disease:
- Nephrologist: This is a physician who is specialized in kidney-related diseases.
- Advanced Practitioner: This is a Physician Assistant (PA) or Nurse Practitioner (NP). These providers work closely with the Nephrologist in providing medical care.
- Nephrology Nurse: This is a Registered Nurse who has undergone additional training and certification to provide care to patients with chronic kidney disease.
- Renal Nutritionist: This is a dietitian who has undergone certification to help meet the nutritional needs of patients with chronic kidney disease.
- Nephrology Social Worker: This professional is a licensed or certified social worker who helps kidney patients and their families obtain the help they need at home. They also coordinate services provided by community agencies to help patients when they are home.
- Renal Technologist: This person works under the nurse and is often the person most directly involved with the patient during dialysis treatments. They often start and end the treatment and monitor the patient throughout.
- Financial Counselor: This person helps the patient and family with questions regarding insurance coverage and patient responsibility for any services provided.

Early referral of ESRD patient to nephrologist

Early referral of the ESRD patient to a nephrologist has been shown to decrease the mortality rate for the ESRD patient. Some of the benefits of early referral of the ESRD patient to a nephrologist include the following:
- Establishment of dietary prescription
- Placement of peritoneal or vascular access
- Timely diagnosis and treatment of hypertension, anemia, phosphatemia, and acidosis

Managing later stages of CKD

The tasks associated with managing the later stages of CKD include preparing the patient for dialysis, determining the best mode of dialysis (outpatient hemodialysis center, peritoneal dialysis, or home hemodialysis) dietary evaluation with phosphorus and volume management, and administration of necessary immunizations. A decision must be made to determine the best course of treatment: either chronic dialysis or renal transplantation.

Emotional impact on patients with chronic kidney disease

Chronic kidney disease, particularly dialysis, has a huge emotional and social impact on patients. Patients on dialysis lose a lot of freedom and their quality of life decreases. It has been widely reported that patients with chronic kidney disease have a higher incidence of depression. It is important that a social support network be intimately involved in the care of all patients with chronic kidney disease. Social workers are extremely important in coordinating home services and addressing family and social issues with all patients.

Stress

Psychosocial aspects that affect the ESRD patient are often associated with stress. Psychosocial issues affect the general health of the ESRD patient. Stress associated with ESRD and dialysis comes from many factors and may have a significant effect on the overall outcome of the treatment. Depression, that may be the result of chronic illness, and a lack of social support have been linked to mortality in numerous studies of ESRD patients. Several of the stressors that affect the ESRD patient include the following:
- Effects of the illness
- Family dynamics
- Dietary restrictions
- Time constraints
- Financial responsibilities
- Functional restraints
- Employment adjustments
- Sexual changes
- Staff interactions
- Personal role modification
- Medication effects
- Concerns regarding life span

National Kidney Foundation

The National Kidney Foundation, Inc. is the major health organization that has established guidelines in the care of patients with kidney diseases. Specifically, the National Kidney Foundation has established the kidney disease outcomes quality initiative (KDOQI). KDOQI provides evidence-based guidelines to all clinicians caring for patients with renal disease. The guidelines include managing anemia in chronic kidney disease, bone metabolism in chronic kidney disease, hemodialysis, peritoneal dialysis, vascular access, nutrition, dyslipidemias, hypertension and antihypertensive therapy, cardiovascular disease in dialysis patients and pediatric bone.

Hemodialysis

Metric system abbreviations

The following are the major abbreviations for the metric system, assuming grams is the unit measure:
- kilo (kg) - 1000 = 10^3
- deka (Dg)– 10 = 10^1
- deci (dg) – 1/10 = 10^{-1}
- centi (cg) – 1/100 = 10^{-2}
- milli (mg) – 1/1000 = 10^{-3}
- micro (µg) – 1/1000000 = 10^{-6}
- nano (ng) - 1/1000000000 = 10^{-9}

Element

Elements are the most fundamental substances in nature. They cannot be broken down into further components without changing their essential properties. They are made up of atoms, which share the same proton number. For example, helium is composed of two protons and exists as a gas naturally. However, if one were to take one proton away from helium, than it would no longer be helium. It would now exist as hydrogen, which is a totally different gas with different properties altogether.

Atom

An atom is the smallest particle of an element that still retains the properties of that element. Atoms are composed of a central nucleus comprised of protons and neutrons with surrounding electrons. The number of protons defines what type of atom it is, e.g. hydrogen has one proton and helium has two protons. Protons have a positive charge and a much larger in comparison to electrons, which have a negative charge. Neutrons are also large particles but they possess neither a positive or negative charge.

Compound

A compound is a combination of different elements. For example, 2 parts hydrogen and one-part oxygen comprise a compound. In contrast, hydrogen and oxygen alone are simply elements. Separately they exist as gases. However, in combination they form water. Compounds can be made of both organic elements (carbon, nitrogen, phosphorus) and inorganic elements (mercury, gold, etc.).

Solution

A solution is a mixture of dissolved particle (solute) into a liquid (solvent). Each solution has different properties based on the solute and solvents used. For example, salt water can be thought of a solution. Sodium Chloride (NaCl) is dissolved in water (H_2O) to form salt water. Be careful not to confuse solutions with compounds. NaCl is one compound and H_2O is another compound. They both retain their properties and the mixture (salt water) does not make a new compound. Understanding solutions is important, particularly with dialysate composition.

Concentration

Concentration is defined as the amount of solute divided by the amount of solvent usually expressed as gm/L. For example, dissolving 1 gram of salt into one liter of water will yield a concentration of 1gm/L. Dissolving 10 grams of salt into one liter of water will yield a concentration of 10gm/L. Intuitively, one can deduce that the latter is more concentrated than the former and thus would taste more salty. Concentrations are important when comprising dialysate solutions and examining blood levels as well.

Ion

An ion is a particle capable of carrying an electric charge. Ions are subdivided according to charge:
- A positively charged ion is called a cation.
- A negatively charged ion is called an anion.

It is also important to remember that ions can be either elements like sodium, which carries a positive charge or compounds like bicarbonate (HCO_3), which carries a negative charge.

Electrolytes

An electrolyte is a substance that dissolves in water to form ions. Ions are particles that carry an electric charge. The most often measured electrolytes include:
- Sodium (Na)
- Potassium (k)
- Chloride (Cl)
- Calcium (Ca)
- Magnesium (Mg)

It is also important to remember that sodium and potassium carry one positive charge (cation). Calcium and magnesium carry two positive charges (cations). Chloride, however, carries one negative charge (anion).

Semipermeable

Semipermeable means allowing the passage of some things while restricting others. For example, dialysis filters are considered semipermeable. That is because they are filters with holes that only permit the passage of certain sized molecules (usually <500 Daltons). Any molecule with a size of greater than 500 Daltons cannot pass through the dialysis filter. Thus, dialysis membranes filter very small molecules such as urea and electrolytes very well. They remove urea from the blood but not more vital elements such as albumin and other proteins.

Osmosis

Osmosis is the movement of fluids from an area of low concentration to an area of high concentration. For example, suppose we place two fluids in the same container separated by a membrane that only allows the passage of fluids. One solution will contain a concentration of 10mg/L of salt (NaCl). The other solution will contain a concentration of 1 mg/L of salt (NaCl). Remember, only fluid is allowed to pass from one part of the container through the membrane (not particles). Because the fluid is more concentrated on the 10mg/L side, fluid will shift from the 1 mg/L side towards the 10mg/L side. Fluid will continue to move until the concentrations on both sides are equal. Another way of looking at it is that there is more fluid on the 1 mg/L side and it will, via osmosis, travel down its concentration gradient towards the 10mg/L.

Diffusion

Diffusion is similar conceptually to osmosis. Osmosis is the movement of *fluids* from an area of low concentration to an area of high concentration, while diffusion is the movement of *particles* from an area of high concentration to low concentration. For example, suppose again that we place two fluids in the same container separated by a membrane that only allows the passage of particles, rather than fluids. One solution will contain a concentration of 10mg/L of salt (NaCl). The other solution will contain a concentration of 1 mg/L of salt (NaCl). Remember, only particles are allowed to pass from one part of the container through the membrane (not fluid). Because the fluid is more concentrated on the 10mg/L side, *particles* will shift down their concentration gradient towards the 1 mg/L side. Particles will continue to move until the concentrations on both sides of the membrane are equal.

Distribution of water in the human body

Total body water can be easily quantified by multiplying body weight by 60%. Thus, the human body is 60% water weight. Yet, how that water is distributed can be subdivided into the following compartments:
- Intravascular
- Interstitial
- Intracellular

Intravascular refers to the water content found in arteries and veins. Interstitial refers to the water content found in capillaries and organs. Intracellular refers to the water content inside the cell only. Most body water is located intracellularly with less in the interstitium and least in the vascular space. Patients with chronic kidney disease may not generate enough urine and thus water balance is disturbed. Hemodialysis patients frequently need excess water removed at each session and the post dialysis weight is commonly referred to as dry weight (weight after dialysis where excess fluid is removed).

Water homeostasis in the average adult

The most important principle in water balance is to understand that a normal adult will take in as much water as he/she will lose. If one takes in excess water, there will be a net positive water balance. If one loses more water, there will be a net negative water balance. The average adult takes in water from ingestion of solids and liquids and from oxidative processes in the body. The total is roughly about 2500 ml. Water is lost through feces, urine and insensible loss. Insensible loss describes water lost via the skin (to cool the body) and via the lungs (with each expiration). If, for example, one exercises, insensible loss via the skin will increase. In order to maintain water balance, the body will trigger thirst sensors and obligate one to drink water. Conversely, if one drinks excess water than one will urinate more to maintain water balance.

Causes of hypotension

Hypotension is most commonly caused by excess water volume removal, antihypertensive medications and acute infections causing sepsis and arrhythmias. Less common causes of hypotension include anaphylaxis, liver cirrhosis and improper blood pressure measurements. In order to differentiate the cause of hypotension, a complete history and physical should be performed prior to any new dialysis patient begins chronic dialysis. Furthermore, any new changes in medical conditions or medications should be duly noted. The sepsis syndrome would be associated with fevers, high white blood cell count and a source of infection (usually access site). Arrhythmias should be suspected if the electrolytes are abnormal and if the pulse rate changes abruptly. Changes in antihypertensive medication dosages frequently lead to hypotension. Anaphylaxis occurs when a severe allergic reaction occurs to a particular food, latex or medicines. Most commonly, an antibiotic is given during dialysis and seconds later the patient is hypotensive. Other signs of an allergic reaction include fevers, hives, and itching. Liver cirrhosis is suggested by history. Poorly measured blood pressures are frequently found with inappropriate cuff sizes, improper placement of the cuff and with automated blood pressure machines.

pH

pH is defined as the negative log of hydrogen ion concentration. It is an indication of the acidity or alkalinity of a solution. The equation is rarely used to compute pH in everyday use but the values are important. Water has a pH of 7.0, which is considered neither an acid nor base. The lower the pH the more acidic a solution becomes. Conversely, the higher the pH the more basic a solution is. The range of acidic levels is between 1.0 – 6.99 and the range for basic solutions is between 7.01 to 14.0. Normal serum pH ranges between 7.35 – 7.45. Understanding pH values is important as it relates to patients with chronic kidney disease. The kidneys are important in filtering and excreting waste. When the waste products accumulate, a total body acidosis ensues. Acidosis is commonly found in patients with chronic kidney disease.

Normal blood flow to kidneys

The kidneys are unique in that 25% of total blood flows from the heart supply the kidneys exclusively. Blood reaches the kidneys through the renal artery. The renal artery then divides into smaller branches until they reach the afferent arteriole. Afferent means carrying towards. The afferent arteriole leads towards the glomerulus, the apparatus where blood is filtered and toxins removed. After the glomerulus, the efferent arteriole carries blood away from the kidneys toward the renal veins (efferent means to carry away). The renal veins carry the blood back towards the heart where the cycle is repeated. The site of action of ace inhibitors is at the efferent arteriole. Be careful not to confuse normal renal blood flow with urine formation. Urine formation is a completely separate process.

Formation of urine

Blood that is filtered at the glomerulus travels through the nephron. The nephron is the mainstay of urine formation.

It is composed of:
- The glomerulus
- Proximal convoluted tubule
- Loop of Henle
- Distal convoluted tubule
- Collecting ducts

The glomerulus is where blood is freely filtered. The proximal convoluted tubule is the site where most reabsorption takes place. For example, bicarbonate is freely filtered in the glomerulus but is largely reabsorbed at the proximal convoluted tubule. The loop of Henle is instrumental in concentrating the urine and reabsorbing electrolytes. The distal convoluted tubule leads towards the collecting ducts where water is reabsorbed to produce concentrated urine. The more water the body needs to retain, the more concentrated the urine will be. Acid and base balance is also regulated by the kidneys at the level of the nephron.

Creatinine

Creatinine is the breakdown product of muscle. Creatinine is useful as a measure of renal function because it is freely filtered and not reabsorbed by the nephrons. Therefore, it is fairly accurate measure of clearance or how well the kidneys clear a substance from the serum. Creatinine is measured in the serum and elevations are indicative of renal failure. However, caution must be taken in using creatinine. Foremost, muscle mass is the most important determinant of creatinine levels. A 300-pound body builder will have a higher creatinine than a 75 year old woman whom has less muscle mass. Furthermore, serum creatinine levels are tougher to interpret in patients with amputations. Therefore, it is imperative to use the Cockcroft-Gault or MDRD equations to accurately assess renal function.

Urea

Urea is the breakdown product of protein metabolism. Proteins are degraded into their component parts by enzymatic reactions and urea is formed as the waste product. Urea is freely filtered at the kidney and is excreted in the urine. When renal failure ensues, urea is not excreted and its levels increase. Urea is measured in the serum as the BUN (blood urea nitrogen). Thus, an indicator for renal failure is an elevated BUN. Moreover, the BUN is used to assess the adequacy of dialysis. Kt/V measures the adequacy of dialysis and the pre- and post-hemodialysis levels of BUN are drawn and factored into the equation.

Albumin

Albumin is the most abundant serum protein in the body. It binds and carries a huge array of compounds including hormones, medications and other proteins. It is also a marker of nutrition. The dialysis patient is at an increased risk of malnutrition. Closely monitoring albumin levels helps the dietitian assess nutritional status. A low albumin level is an indicator of malnutrition and has been associated with increased hospitalization and slower recovery from infections. However, caution must be taken when interpreting albumin levels. A normal albumin does not necessarily indicate proper nutrition. In fact, many dialysis patients have normal albumin levels and remain malnourished.

Fluid shifts in the body during dialysis

Fluid is removed from the body via ultrafiltration. The fluid that is removed comes from the intravascular space. In order to compensate for the intravascular hypovolemia, fluid shifts from the interstitial and intracellular spaces into the blood stream. If the rate of fluid removal (ultrafiltration rate) is too high, fluid will be removed faster than it can be replaced from the interstitium. This will result in hypotension and patients can go into shock. The best method of preventing hypotension is to control the ultrafiltration rate with frequent blood pressure monitoring during dialysis. Furthermore, should hypotension occur, intravenous hypertonic saline could be administered. The hypertonicity will force fluid via osmosis to shift from the interstitial and intracellular spaces into the vasculature. The hypertonic saline would not necessarily correct the hypovolemia directly but will assist in proper fluid shifting.

Biocompatibility

Biocompatibility refers to the body's response when blood interacts with the dialyzer membrane. The dialyzer membrane is a foreign substance. When blood comes into contact with the dialyzer, it will react as if it is being invaded by activating the immune system. The immune system will trigger complement activation (proteins found in the body which activate a cascade of reactions resulting in an immunologic defense). Complement is also a marker for inflammation. The chronic inflammation and complement activation is hazardous to patients and the former is being closely studied today. Cellulose based membranes are less biocompatible than synthetic membranes. The reason synthetic membranes are more biocompatible is that they have fewer antigens on their surface, which the blood recognizes as foreign.

Hemodialysis

History of dialysis

The history of "dialysis" began when the London chemist, Thomas Graham, first coined the term in 1861. He gave this name to the process of selective diffusion. In 1913, Abel, Rowntree, and Turner developed a device which utilized collodion tubes through which blood poured while a saline solution washed over the outside of the tubes. This apparatus was implemented successfully in treating animals with uremia. Kolff and Berk later developed an artificial kidney, using the newly developed anticoagulant, heparin and cellophane tubing. In 1948, Skeggs and Leonards invented a parallel plate dialyzer. The first disposable dialyzer, the Travenol twin coil unit, came on the market in 1956. Gambro started production of the disposable parallel plate devices in 1965. Hollow-fiber artificial kidneys were invented at around this same time in the United States.

Hemodialysis

Hemodialysis refers to the process of removing or filtering metabolic wastes out of the blood through a semipermeable membrane. The goal is to supplement the normal functioning of a kidney by managing uremia, fluid overload, and electrolyte imbalance. Molecular size is measured in daltons (DA). Many of the substances that cause uremia have a dalton size of less than 500. These molecules easily diffuse across the cellulose membranes. Particles larger than 500 DA (midsize molecules) diffuse inadequately through these membranes. Large molecules (more than 3000 DA) are not commonly thought to be toxic, except for β_2 microglobulin because of its relationship with bone disease, amyloid, and anemia.

Dialyzers

There are two main types of dialyzers: parallel plate and hollow fiber. The parallel plate dialyzers work by putting membranes in layers, one on top of the other. The membranes are not flat but are curved with ridges to expand the surface area. The main drawbacks of parallel plate dialyzers are the inability for reuse and compliance (the higher the transmembrane pressure, the higher the volume of blood held). Thus, ultrafiltration cannot be controlled very precisely. The other type of dialyzer is the hollow fiber or HFAK (hollow fiber artificial kidney). This is the most common type of dialyzer used today. It woks by having hollow fibers arranged in bundles. They can come in different sizes and thickness and are made of either cellulose or are synthetic. The main advantages of HFAK include being noncompliant and reuse.

High efficiency and high flux dialysis

High efficiency dialysis refers to cellulosic membranes with increased surface areas. High flux dialysis refers to synthetic membranes with increased surface areas and permeability to larger molecules. The advantage of high flux membranes is their decreased association with cardiovascular events. They also clear β2 microglobulin more efficiently and produce less inflammation by activating complement. They have also been shown to increase patient survival after long-term dialysis treatment (>3.7 years as per the HEMO study). The main problem with high flux dialyzers is that the increased permeability allows for easier access to the patient's bloodstream by gram-negative bacteria.

Arteriovenous hemodialysis and venovenous hemodialysis

CAVHD and CVVHD remove solutes and fluid via diffusion. The former uses arterial blood pressure to supply the forces needed to drive blood through the extracorporeal circuit. The latter relies on an external blood pump for flow. A dialysate is used which allows solutes to diffuse down the concentration gradients. Relative to CAVH or CVVH, fluid removal is less efficient. However, solute removal is much better.

Arteriovenous and venovenous techniques

Arteriovenous requires both an arterial line and venous line. Arterial blood leaves the body and enters the dialyzer. Blood travels through the dialysis machine under the body's blood pressure. Note that there are no blood pumps providing negative pressure to aid the passage of blood as it travels through the dialyzer. Finally, blood returns to the body via a venous line. Venovenous, on the other hand, only requires a venous line. Blood leaves the body and enters the dialysis machine. However, a blood pump is required to aid the passage of blood. This is because the venous system is a low-pressure system. Blood returns to the body via another lumen into the same large vein.

Advantages and disadvantages
The major advantage to arteriovenous access is its lack of dependence on a blood pump for filtration. This is very important because the patient's blood pressure is supplying the forces of forward flow. A blood pump applies a negative pressure to entice forward flow. The blood pump places the patient at risk for hypotension during the treatment session. The advantage of a venovenous system is that only one vein needs to be punctured for renal replacement and requires less systemic anticoagulation.

The disadvantage of an arteriovenous system includes more anticoagulation, the puncturing of an artery and less reliable blood flow. Again, blood flow is completely reliant on the patient's blood pressure, which can be low in critically ill patients. The disadvantage of a venovenous system is the use of a blood pump (greater chance of hypotension).

Continuous arteriovenous hemofiltration and continuous venovenous hemofiltration

CAVH and CVVH remove solutes and fluid via convection. The former uses arterial blood pressure to supply the forces needed to drive blood through the extracorporeal circuit. The latter relies on an external blood pump for flow. Both operate by removing fluid and solute via convection with replacement fluids to replace excess fluid loss. These techniques are extremely inefficient requiring treatment sessions of up to 24 hours sometimes.

Purification of dialysis solution

Dialysis solution must meet purification standards to avoid patient injury. 120-200 L of dialysis solution comes in direct contact with the patient's blood during dialysis. Small molecular weight contaminants would have access to the bloodstream, possibly causing chemical or microbiologic injury. A purification system must be employed if municipal water is to be used for dialysis. Common contaminants that may be found in water are as follows:
- Aluminum: may cause bone disease, fatal neurologic deterioration, dialysis encephalopathy syndrome, and anemia
- Chloramine: hemolytic anemia
- Fluoride: severe pruritus, nausea, and fatal ventricular fibrillation
- Copper and zinc: hemolytic anemia
- Bacteria and endotoxins: may cause infections and pyrogenic reactions

Quality of dialysis water supply

Meticulous procedures including thorough documentation of the performance of every section of the distribution system must be observed. Standards developed by the AAMI and the European Best Practices Group should be followed in order to maintain optimal patient safety. These include the following:
- Monitor chemical purity of water and dialysis solution.
- Check chloramine levels daily.
- Take chronic toxic component readings in feed water on a regular schedule.
- Measure bacterial growth and endotoxins in water and dialysis fluid using high sensitivity methods.
- Monitor patients for hemolytic, pyrogenic, other reactions, and blood aluminum levels.

A water supply that meets all the standards for the Safe Drinking Water Act and the EPA standards is still not safe for dialysis use. Tap water may be acidic or alkaline, causing problems with the bicarbonate mode of the delivery system maintaining the proper pH. Any contaminants in the water could enter the patient's bloodstream through the dialysis membrane. Substances that may be harmless when water is ingested through the GI system could be toxic if absorbed directly into the blood. Tap water may contain chemicals, organic compounds, nonionic organic compounds, silt, pesticides, herbicides, minerals, microorganisms, trace elements, and endotoxins not found in high-purity water approved for dialysis. The dialyzer membrane cannot distinguish between ions to be absorbed or rejected, making it necessary to eliminate these contaminants prior to their introduction into the dialysis process.

There are many organic and inorganic impurities found in tap water, including chemical solutes, bacteria and their by-products, and particulate matter. Some of the chemicals that can be found in tap water that can be harmful to human beings if found in excess are as follows:
- Chloramines and nitrates: may cause methemoglobinemia in which red blood cells no longer have the ability to carry oxygen
- Copper: may cause hemolysis
- Manganese: toxicity

- Iron: toxicity
- Fluoride: accumulates in bone, aggravates uremic bone disease, toxic to enzyme systems
- Aluminum: accumulates, is related to dialysis-dementia syndrome, anemia and osteodystrophy
- Zinc: GI upset and anemia
- 90Sr: radioactive, poses health danger

Routine tests to assure safety of water treatment system

Routine tests that are done on water treatment systems are as follows:
- Conductivity testing is conducted to assure that the feed and product water contains the proper amount of ions. This is done with a Phoenix meter or a Myron-1.
- Bacterial culturing is done to identify any growth in the water or dialysate.
- Resistivity testing is performed to determine the effectiveness of the deionizer.
- Hardness testing determines the amount of calcium and magnesium.
- The total dissolved solids (TDS) measurement verifies the efficiency of the reverse osmosis system by measuring the sum of all the ions in the solution.

Treatment of water in preparation for hemodialysis

Below are ways through which water is treated in preparation for hemodialysis:
- Filtration
- Activated carbon filters (adsorption)
- Water softeners
- Reverse osmosis
- Deionization
- Ultraviolet light exposure

Role of water softeners
The term "water softener" refers to removing calcium and magnesium from the water supply. Thus, "hard water" is water with too much calcium and magnesium. The water softener works by exchanging sodium ions for both calcium and magnesium. The exchange is two sodium for one calcium and two sodium for one magnesium (recall that sodium carries one positive charge and calcium and magnesium are divalent cations). The removal of calcium and magnesium is important in preparing the water prior to further treatment. Other positively charged ions are also removed by the water softener including aluminum.

Role of carbon tanks
The carbon tank functions to purify water via activated carbon. The activated carbon helps remove chlorines, chloramines and organic matter via adsorption. There are two carbon tanks at each dialysis facility.
- The first tank is a high flow state that removes most of the chlorine and chloramines.
- The second tank is a low flow state to get any remaining chlorines. The low flow state is more conducive to bacterial growth. Thus, dialysis facilities change the order of tank use daily. Moreover, at the end of each day the tanks must be backwashed so that they can effectively filter the next day. The carbon tanks can be changed entirely by an outside vendor to ensure filter integrity periodically. However, some tanks need not be changed but simply have the carbon filter changed at regular intervals.

Role of deionization
Deionization is the process of removing all ions from the water supply. Both cations and anions are removed so that the water used is nonconductive. The process of cation removal involves exchanging hydrogen ions for the cations involved (mostly sodium, potassium, calcium and magnesium). The process of anion removal involves exchanging hydroxide (usually exchanged with chloride, fluoride, sulfate and nitrate). The combination of hydrogen and hydroxide ions combine to form water. However, the major drawback to deionization is that it does not remove endotoxins. Thus, following deionization, a filter or reverse osmosis is needed to remove endotoxins.

Role of reverse osmosis
Reverse osmosis is important in freeing water from any leftover contaminants following carbon tanks and water softeners. The water is placed under a high pressure system and is filtered via a semipermeable membrane. The high pressure is needed to ensure that most contaminants, including endotoxins, are picked up while water is forced through the membrane. The water that is emerges is extremely pure and will be held before use for hemodialysis. Reverse osmosis is also referred to as ultrafiltration of the water system. This is not to be confused with the ultrafiltration that occurs during dialysis (removal of excess water from patient's plasma). Rather, this is ultrafiltration at the level of water preparation prior to dialysis treatment.

Role of ultraviolet light
Ultraviolet light is used to destroy bacteria contained in water. The light passes through the water and damages the DNA structure of bacteria. It effectively destroys bacteria but does not affect endotoxin. The limitations of ultraviolet light are a need for a low flow state and clarity of water. A low flow state is needed so that the light can effectively penetrate the water. Also, cloudy water distorts ultraviolet light and can lessen its efficacy in eliminating bacteria.

Preparation of dialyzer for use

Foremost, all dialyzers must be clean of any matter or bacteria when it is received from the manufacturer. The dialyzer should be washed saline solution to clear any leftover particulates. It must also be washed with disinfectant to rid it of any bacteria. Second, it must be free of any air. Air trapped in the dialyzer could easily diffuse into the patient's blood stream and cause an air embolism. Air can also clog the hollow fiber filters and render them ineffective.

Priming the dialyzer

New and reused dialyzers have to be primed using 500-1000 mL of normal saline solution, depending on the type of unit. All manufacturers have instructions on how to prime their particular dialyzers. Their recommendations should be read and meticulously followed. New units may contain glycerin and particulates that remained from the manufacturing method and will require 1000 mL of saline to ensure that all the contaminants are removed. 500 mL of saline should be sufficient for priming a reused unit with the primer flowing in a counterclockwise pathway to remove any remaining disinfectant.

Removing air from the dialyzer

All air needs to be removed from the dialyzer beginning at the bottom. Attach the bloodlines to the dialyzer; turn the dialyzer venous side up and prime with normal saline solution. Next, use the arterial bloodline; infuse the normal saline solution through the dialyzer and out the venous bloodline into a container. As the dialyzer is filled with saline, air will be forced up and out the top. Gently tap the dialyzer and turn it side to side to ensure that all the air is completely out of the header.

Types of membranes used in dialyzers

Don't confuse the type of membranes with type of dialyzers. Parallel and hollow fibers only describe the contour of the membranes and not their composition. Membranes are composed of either cellulose or synthetic. Cellulose is a carbohydrate polymer that is found in plants. It is manufactured to form different thickness and water absorptive qualities and permeabilites. The most common cellulose membrane is cuprophan. The other type of membrane used is synthetically manufactured. The most common types include polyacrylonitrile, polysulfone, polyamide and polymehtyl-methacrylate. They are all easily reused and are noncompliant.

Synthetic membranes

Synthetic membranes for hemodialysis are thermoplastics, which feature fine, smooth, luminal surfaces sustained by a spongy wall structure. Varieties include polyacrylonitrile (PAN), Polysulfone (P_4S) polyamide, poly-methacrylate (PMMA), and others. Convective transfer accounts for their mass transport.

Advantages of the synthetic membrane are as follows:
- Reusability
- Bioincompatibility

Disadvantages of synthetic membranes include the following:
- Expensive in comparison to cellulose membranes
- High water permeability-ultrafiltration needs to be used
- Absorption of protein to the membrane surface
- Risk of reverse filtration from dialysate to blood

Cellulose membranes

Cellulose membranes are comprised of a naturally occurring substance. However, that does not necessitate any advantage. Cellulose is cheaper to manufacture and have been in use for a long time. The characteristics of cellulose membranes are better studied than synthetic membranes. However, they cannot be reused and are somewhat bioincompatible (cause an inflammatory response).

Mass transfer rate

Mass transfer rate refers to the rate of transfer of solutes across a semipermeable membrane. In dialysis, mass transfer rate applies to the rate of transfer (removal) of toxins and electrolytes, particularly urea and potassium. The mass transfer rate is affected by:
- Temperature
- Surface area of the semipermeable membrane
- Concentration gradient
- Membrane permeability
- Blood
- Dialysate flow rates and flow geometry (usually countercurrent flow)

Mass transfer rates are increased with higher temperatures, greater membrane surface areas and higher concentration gradients.

Countercurrent flow

Countercurrent flow exists when one fluid is passing in one direction while another fluid is passing in the opposite direction. What separates the two fluids is a semipermeable membrane. In dialysis, blood from the patient flows continuously in one direction while the dialysate solution flows in the opposite direction. The fluids do not intermix and are separated by a semipermeable membrane. The fluids travel in opposite direction to maintain the difference in concentration gradients in the dialyzer. Imagine if both blood and dialysate started at one end of the dialyzer and flowed in the same direction. As they reached the end of the dialyzer the concentration of urea and other electrolytes would equilibrate. However, if the fluids traveled in opposite directions, equilibration would not occur. Urea and other toxins would constantly diffuse from the blood into the dialysate solution down their concentration gradients for the length of the dialyzer.

Physiologic importance
Countercurrent flow is important in removing toxins and electrolytes from the blood. It allows for a continuous concentration gradient to exist. For example, urea is highly concentrated in blood. As the blood passes through the dialyzer it meets the dialysate solution coming in the opposite direction. Dialysate has a lower urea concentration and thus urea will travel from the blood into the dialysate. The countercurrent flow creates an environment where urea is constantly diffusing down its concentration gradient. The exact same physiology occurs in the kidney where excess toxins and electrolytes are removed in the nephron.

Ultrafiltration

Ultrafiltration refers to hydrostatic pressures forcing plasma volume out of the blood and into the dialysate. Another term for ultrafiltration is transmembrane pressure. Ultrafiltration occurs as follows:
- Blood is delivered to the dialyzer under positive pressure.
- This hydrostatic pressure forces some volume of blood to traverse the semipermeable membrane into the dialysate solution.
- Moreover, dialysate is traveling under negative pressure.
- The negative pressure accentuates the removal of fluid.

It is via ultrafiltration that patients lose the excess water gained between dialysis sessions.

Ultrafiltration controls

Ultrafiltration controls are used to match the volume of dialysate entering the dialyzer with the volume of dialysate emerging from the dialyzer plus water from the patient. Under normal circumstances, the ultrafiltration will be such that there should be more volume leaving the dialyzer than that entering the dialyzer (recall ultrafiltration is the process of removing excess water from the patient). Parameters are set to the ultrafiltration to govern control of too much or too little volume being removed. There are two types of controls:
- Volumetric
- Flowmetric

Volumetric and flowmetric ultrafiltration controls
Volumetric ultrafiltration works by a diaphragm system. As dialysate passes the first diaphragm, an equal volume is delivered to the dialyzer. Than a second diaphragm detects dialysate as it emerges from the dialyzer. As fluid emerges from the dialyzer, an equal volume is delivered to the drain. Flowmetric ultrafiltration works by having detectors of fluid flow in both the inflow and outflow dialysate pathways. Fluid balance is monitored and controlled through the flowmetric monitors.

Isolated ultrafiltration

Isolated ultrafiltration refers to removal of water without solute. The patient is hooked up to the dialysis machine and blood flows through the dialyzer. However, no dialysate is used during the process. Thus, there is little to no solute loss. However, hydrostatic forces are still at play and water is removed from the patient. Ultrafiltration is indicated in patients which are volume overloaded but do not need solute removal i.e. urea, potassium.

Reverse filtration

Reverse filtration is just the opposite of ultrafiltration. Instead of blood passing under positive pressure and dialysate under negative pressure, the opposite occurs. Now dialysate is under positive pressure while blood is under negative pressure. The danger with reverse filtration is that patients will gain fluid instead of losing it. They will also take on other substances in the dialysate solution such as bicarbonate, potassium and possibly infectious agents (bacteria). Reverse filtration is usually identified via an alarm on the dialysis machine. Dialysis must be immediately stopped if reverse filtration is detected.

Recirculation

Recirculation occurs when blood coming from the dialysis machine is returned to the dialyzer. The arterial systemic circulation should enter the dialyzer and return to the venous side. However, if blood returning from the dialyzer is again circulated back to the dialysis machine, recirculation is taking place. The way to identify recirculation is to obtain an arterial sample from the systemic side and a sample from the arterial line headed towards the dialysis machine. The concentrations of urea should be the same in both samples. If, however, the arterial line has a lower urea concentration than the systemic arterial sample than recirculation is present. Well functioning fistulas should have a recirculation percentage of below 10 percent.

Factors that affect blood resistance as it flows through the dialysis machine

The number one factor affecting blood resistance is the patient's hematocrit. Hematocrit is the main determinant of blood viscosity. The larger the hematocrit, the more viscous and more resistance to blood flow. The other factor in determining blood resistance is the path blood takes as it travels through the dialyzer. The longer the dialyzer the more resistance blood will encounter. The larger the surface area and cross sectional area of the dialyzer, the lower the resistance. These are basic principles of fluid mechanics and a more detailed explanation is provided by Bernoulli's principles. However, for purposes of flow resistance in dialysis the important points to remember are hematocrit and dialyzer length, surface and cross sectional areas.

Hemodialysis and hemofiltration

Hemodialysis is the removal of water and solute via diffusion. Blood enters the dialyzer with dialysate flowing in a countercurrent fashion. Solutes diffuse down there concentration gradient from blood to dialysate (removal of urea and potassium). Conversely, calcium and bicarbonate diffuse down their concentration gradient from dialysate to blood. In contrast, hemofiltration does not use diffusion at all. It removes water and solute via convective forces. Dialysate is not used for this technique. Blood enters the dialyzer and small solutes and water are removed under hydrostatic pressure. In order to prevent excess water loss, replacement fluid is needed for hemofiltration. The fluid replacement aids in diluting lost solutes such as urea and potassium and thus their serum levels decrease.

CRRT

Continuous renal replacement therapy (CRRT) is a generic term that applies to various techniques. It operates by removing water and solute via diffusion (dialysis based solute removal) or convection (filtration based solute removal). It is a continuous process and is referred to as a "slow dialysis." There are many techniques in carrying out CRRT and they are essentially categorized based on access. CRRT variations include:
- Slow continuous ultrafiltration (SCUF)
- Continuous arteriovenous hemofiltration (CAVH)
- Continuous arteriovenous hemodialysis (CAVHD)
- Continuous venovenous hemofiltration (CVVH)
- Continuous venovenous hemodialysis (CVVHD)

For CAVH and CAVHD, arterial access is required. For all others there is no need for arterial access as double lumen catheters are placed in large veins. However, CVVH and CVVHD require a blood pump during the procedure.

Blood pump readings

Blood pumps that have rate indicators display the flow determined by the speed of rotation. The variables that could affect the accuracy of the blood pump's readings are as follows:
- Internal diameter of tubing: must match that which was used for calibrating the pump
- Pressure conditions in blood circuit
- Lack of linearity across indicator scale
- Type of tubing used

The calibration process should be done on a regular basis, under standard conditions, with the exact brand and lot of tubing that is being used clinically. The water used should be at 37° C, pumped from the source through partially clamped tubing to approximate the negative pressure between the needle and the dialysis pump. A graduated cylinder should be used for holding the outflow solution, and it should be collected over a 3 to 5 minute period. The resulting volume in millimeters divided by the time in minutes gives the flow rate.

Ultrasonic air/foam detector

The ultrasonic air/foam detector is a commonly used type of apparatus for detection the presence of air. It uses ultrasonic beams to find air, foam, or microbubbles in the blood. Since sound traverses liquid more rapidly than air, even minute levels of air will disrupt the sonic beam and trigger the alarm. The alarm system of most ultrasonic detectors may be disarmed while priming and rinsing the dialysis delivery system. When the alarm system is inactive, a constant, low-level alarm should be sounding, to indicate the disarmed state. Dialysis should never be performed on a patient when the air/foam detector is not activated.

Blood leak monitors

Blood leaks occur when blood traverses the semipermeable membrane and flows with the dialysate. As dialysate leaves the dialyzer it passes over a light sensor. If the light is obstructed from reaching its sensor via a change in fluid composition (i.e. blood), than an alarm sounds. Locating where the blood leak occurs is crucial and dialysis is temporarily halted. Obviously, blood leaking into the system will have serious effects on the patient including hypotension, electrolyte imbalance and possibly death.

Dialyzer reuse

Dialyzer reuse is the process of sterilizing the dialyzer after it is used. Dialyzer reuse is authorized for the same patient only. For infection control purposes, dialyzers are not allowed to be cleaned and reused on different patients. The main advantage of reuse is lower costs and fewer first pass side effects (each dialyzer is different and each time one is introduced, patients may experience side effects).

The disadvantages of reuse include:
- Expensive sterilizing techniques
- Hazardous sterilizing materials and chemicals
- Quality control to ensure proper dialyzer storage and to ensure it is reused in the same patient only

The following are the four main criteria used to determine dialyzer reusability:
- Total cell volume – most common method to determine dialyzer reusability. The dialyzer is initially filled with water and than emptied (before being used on a patient). Than after hemodialysis the dialyzer is again filled with water and emptied. The emptied water must measure at least 80% of the initial water volume. If it is less than eighty percent, the dialyzer is not fit for reuse.
- Pressure testing – also referred to as leak testing. This test ensures there is no blood leak during dialysis. Pressure is applied to the dialyzer. If the pressure falls, than there is a leak and the dialyzer is not fit for use.

- Ultrafiltration coefficient – used as an indirect measure of how well dialyzers clear substances. This is not to be confused with clearance but rather a test of the membrane's permeability.
- Visual inspection – Examining the dialyzer for large blood streaks indicates clotted membranes and not fit for use.

The process in cleaning a dialyzer prior to reuse is described below:
- The dialyzer is first flushed with saline to remove left over blood products.
- Then a cleanser is added to clear all contaminants including bacteria.
- After cleaning and disinfecting, the dialyzer is tested for integrity of use. The membrane must still be intact and capable of removing waste.
- Finally, a disinfectant is used as a final step to clear all contaminants and waste.

SDS

The method used to deliver solutions used to produce dialysate to the machine is called the SDS, or solution delivery system. The overhead holding tank is referred to as the "head" tank. Bicarbonate from a mixing tank and acid from a storage tank are transferred to the head tank. These solutions are gravity fed to a solution distribution system (SDS) and then routed to the treatment area where it enters a series of pipes attached to the dialysis machines. Some supply only one patient while other solution delivery systems supply several dialyzers at the same time.

Dialysate

Dialysate is a solution, prepared as a chemical composition, to be as similar to normal plasma as possible. It carries away waste materials and excess fluid extracted from the blood by the dialysis process. Dialysate prevents the depletion of essential electrolytes and prevents the removal of excess water. The five chemicals that are most frequently used to make dialysate are as follows:
- Sodium chloride
- Sodium bicarbonate or sodium acetate
- Calcium chloride
- Potassium chloride
- Magnesium chloride

In some cases, glucose is also added to the formulation.

Primary and secondary tests to assure the composition of dialysate

The primary test calculates the concentration of a solute by the laboratory method called reliability. Two such tests are flame photometry for testing sodium content and titration to find chloride. This type of analysis is important to assure the proper ratio of acid to bicarbonate and to determine the ratio of concentrate to water. The secondary test uses overall conductivity. Most suppliers of concentrate indicate on the label the proper level of conductivity that should be seen when the solution is properly mixed. Another secondary test measures total osmolality by freezing-point depression or vapor pressure to determine the total amount of solute in the dialysate.

Proportioning systems

Proportioning systems, most of which use microprocessor circuitry to control the pace of the proportioning pumps and the volume of concentrates added, ensure that the dialysis fluid is properly mixed. The advantages of the proportioning systems are as follows:
- These systems mix fixed volumes of dialysate concentrates with fixed volumes of heated purified water or use conductivity-based servo control systems to mix the concentrates and water.
- Ionic composition of the final dialysate is checked by conductivity.
- If the conductivity is outside the proper range, alarms sound and dialysis stops.

The main disadvantages of proportioning systems are as follows:
- Expense of the units
- Preprogrammed functions may be difficult to change
- Sensors and monitoring devices must reliable and redundant
- Difficult to troubleshoot
- May need factory representative for repairs

Deaeration devices

Deaeration devices are used on dialysate solution. Water from a public water source is below room temperature and needs to be heated before being delivered to the dialyzer, usually at 35°-38° C. Microbubbles and dissolved air are found in water. As the temperature increases, the air trapped in the water is released as expanding microbubbles. These microbubbles negatively affect conductivity sensors, temperature and flowmeters. These bubbles also diminish the contact of the dialysate and membrane in hollow-fiber dialyzers. To release the dissolved air from the solution, deaeration devices use a combination of heat and negative pressure. These air bubbles are trapped by a coalescing filter then vented to the outside.

"A" and "B" concentrate

The "A" concentrate contains a high level of sodium, along with calcium, magnesium, potassium, chloride, and a minimal amount of acetic acid. The "B" (bicarbonate) concentrate is made of the sodium bicarbonate. In some systems, a portion of the sodium chloride is mixed into this solution to increase its overall conductivity, producing a concentrate that is simple to monitor. In the proportioning system, the "B" concentrate is frequently diluted with water, while the "A" concentrate is then mixed in and the resulting fluid flows into the dialyzer. In the closed system, CO_2 is unable to be released as bubbles; therefore, the reaction between the sodium bicarbonate and the acetic acid cannot come to fruition, and the hydrogen ion content keeps the calcium in solution.

SVS

The sodium variation system (SVS), also known as sodium modeling, is a device that may be instituted to decrease some of the complications of hemodialysis treatment, specifically, cramping and hypotension. In rapid dialysis, the fluid is depleted from the intravascular space, and the replenishing of this fluid may not happen quickly enough to prevent hypotension. When the blood pressure falls, cramping of the arms and legs occurs due to their decreased vascular volume. Hypoalbuminemia and right-sided heart failure may also play a part in the delayed refilling of this fluid. The SVS uses a computer model of sodium and water movement between compartments during the hemodialysis procedure. The sodium content varies during the treatment by either adding a special NaCl concentrate or by varying the proportion of the usual concentrate.

Sorbent regenerative system

The sorbent regenerative system uses a cartridge of absorbent materials through which dialysate is recirculated and chemically regenerated. This process removes metabolic wastes from the dialysate and the pH and electrolyte content are restored. This system performs these actions:
- Converts urea to ammonium carbonate
- Absorbs creatinine and other nonionized solutes
- Ion exchange resins (sodium zirconium phosphate and zirconium oxide)

The contents of the four chambers of the sorbent regenerative cartridge are as follows:
- Activated carbon
- Hydrated zirconium oxide
- Zirconium phosphate
- Urease

Advantages and disadvantages
The advantages of the sorbent system are as follows:
- Portability
- No need for special water supply
- No need for special drainage connections
- Adaptable to various electrical systems

The disadvantages of the sorbent system are as follows:
- Expensive cartridge
- Limit on capacity to eliminate urea
- Limit on capacity to absorb ammonia
- Ammonia may build-up in the system and in the patient
- Large patients with high urea levels may need additional cartridge

Additional equipment needed during dialysis
The additional equipment needed for dialysis includes the following:
- Blood pump with blood flow rate
- Heparin infusion pump
- Air/foam detector
- Inflow and outflow pressure sensors

Bicarbonate

Bicarbonate dialysate is the standard of practice in most dialysis facilities. The diffusion of bicarbonate acts as a buffer to the hydrogen ions during hemodialysis and aids in the acid-base balance. Since one of the goals of hemodialysis is to correct acidosis associated with renal failure, sodium bicarbonate concentrate is added to the dialysate as one of the three streams of fluid used. The concentrate comes packaged in two sections. One is "acid concentrate" and the other is "bicarbonate concentrate".

The three streams of fluid are as follows:
- Water, 34 parts
- Acid concentrate, 1 part
- Bicarbonate concentrate, 1.8 parts

Different types of equipment use concentrates of varying compositions. Mismatched concentrate may lead to a fatal error.

Dialysate solution function

Dialysate solution functions to remove urea, certain electrolytes and other wastes from the blood. It must also ensure to not remove other electrolytes or excess water. It accomplishes this by being near identical to serum in its electrolyte concentrations. Dialysate is mostly composed of the following: sodium chloride, sodium bicarbonate or sodium acetate, calcium chloride, potassium chloride and magnesium chloride. Most concentrations of these solutions are standard with the exception of potassium chloride. The potassium concentration is dictated with the dialysis orders based on serum potassium levels. Higher serum potassium will necessitate greater removal and thus a lower potassium dialysate concentration.

Monitoring dialysate concentration

Dialysate concentration is monitored by the conductivity monitor. The conductivity monitor senses total electrolyte or ion flow in the dialysate solution. The conductivity monitor cannot sense individual electrolyte concentrations (e.g. Na concentration of dialysate). However, it can detect total electrolyte flow. Conductivity monitors essentially function just like batteries with monitoring occurring as electrolytes flow past them. Just like batteries, over time they run out and must be replaced. The purpose of conductivity is to ensure that electrical current is not circulating through the dialysis apparatus and transferred to the patient.

Controlling dialysate temperature

Foremost, dialysate temperature should be kept at near normal body temperature. A cold dialysate can cause hypothermia for the patient. Conversely, a hot dialysate can cause hypotension and hemolysis. During dialysis water is removed causing a hypovolemia. The body's natural response is to vasoconstrict to maintain blood pressure. If the dialysate is too warm, the body's ability to vasoconstrict is limited and hypotension ensues. Also, hot dialysate can lead to hemolysis, which can persist for hours. The temperature of the dialysate is set and monitored by the machine and should be kept at around 36 degrees Celsius.

LAL test

LAL is short for limulus amebocyte lysate. It is a test of the water dialysate to check for endotoxins. Endotoxins are found with gram-negative bacteria. Because the water system used for dialysate is not sterile, gram-negative bacteria can contaminate the water. Dialysate with gram-negative bacteria can lead to severe complications including sepsis and patient death. The LAL test is performed daily to ensure the water system is negative for bacteria.

Factors that affect removal of toxins

During dialysis, there are several factors that affect the successful removal of toxins. Six of the factors that affect the successful removal of toxins are as follows:
- Temperature of the dialysate: higher temperature = more solutes removed
- Flow rate: faster dialysate flow rate = greater removal of solutes
- Molecular weight of solutes: lower molecular weight = more solute removal
- Concentration gradient: higher concentration = higher diffusion
- Membrane permeability: more permeable membrane = greater removal of solutes
- Blood flow rate: greater blood flow = greater removal of solutes

The term semipermeable membrane refers to a membrane that allows certain substances to filter through while separating out others. Large molecules are retained in the membrane while smaller molecules easily traverse.

Viscosity of the blood

Hematocrit levels affect the viscosity (thickness and stickiness) of the blood. The greater the number of RBC's in the blood, the higher the hematocrit level. Centipoise is the term used to measure the viscosity of a liquid. Blood with a 30% hematocrit level is around 2.5 centipoise, or about 2.5 times as viscous as water.

Geometry aspects of blood pathway

The "geometric" properties of the blood pathway are the physical properties, such as length, width, surfaces, cross-sections, etc. Geometric aspects include the following:
- The length of the pathway is important, short pathways (15-50 cm) as in the hollow-fiber dialyzers offer low resistance.
- The number of pathways affect the resistance, the higher the number, the lower the resistance, e.g. hollow-fiber dialyzers with thousands of pathways have very low resistance.

The cross-sectional area of a pathway plays a significant role; the larger the cross-sectional pathway, the lower the amount of resistance. In hollow-fiber dialyzers, the internal radius is the control factor.

Initiating hemodialysis in patients without Chronic Kidney Disease Stage V

The following are reasons for initiating hemodialysis in patients who do not have Chronic Kidney Disease Stage V:
- Volume overload
- Metabolic acidosis
- Uremic Encephalopathy
- Refractory Hypertension
- Hyperkalemia
- Hyper or Hypocalcemia
- Pericarditis
- Ingestion of dialyzable products

Complications

The most common complications that occur during dialysis treatment are as follows:
- Hypotension
- Cramping
- Nausea and vomiting
- Headache
- Chest pain
- Back pain
- Itching
- Fever and chills

Dry weight

The term "dry weight" refers to the postdialysis weight at which the patient has had all of his or her excess body fluid removed. If the measurement of dry weight is set too high, the patient will continue to be in a fluid-overloaded state after the dialysis treatment. This could result in edema or pulmonary congestion. If the number is too low, the patient may experience hypotension in the latter part of the dialysis treatment and complain of cramping, dizziness, and malaise after the treatment is complete.

Acute renal failure in pediatric patients

Special considerations must be given to children undergoing hemodialysis. The pediatric dialysis nurse needs to have a thorough understanding of pediatric nursing plus childhood growth and development. In addition, a comprehensive knowledge of the causes of both acute renal failure and chronic renal failure is imperative. Some of the most common causes for acute renal failure in the pediatric patient include the following:
- Septic shock - resulting in hypoperfusion of the kidneys
- Hypotension - causing hypoperfusion of the kidneys
- Severe dehydration - from gastroenteritis or acute blood loss from surgery or an accident, also results in hypoperfusion
- Acute tubular necrosis - from nephrotoxic drugs such as aminoglycoside, antibiotics, and amphotericin B
- Hemolytic uremic syndrome - most common cause of acute renal failure in children in North America

Although acute poststreptococcal glomerulonephritis is frequently seen in the pediatric population, it rarely results in the need for dialysis.

Comorbid conditions that can complicate ESRD treatment in patients

Comorbid conditions in the elderly dialysis patients that complicate treatment for ESRD include the following:
- Cardiovascular disease
- Diabetes
- Reduced protein intake and delayed protein synthesis
- Osteoporosis
- Pulmonary disease

- Impaired vision
- Poor mobility
- Cognition difficulties
- Lack of coordination
- Socioeconomic and psychosocial issues/although not physical, complicate treatment

Advantages of in-center treatment for older patients

Advantages of in-center hemodialysis for the elderly patient are numerous and consist of the following:
- Social interaction with dialysis personnel
- Frequent observation by medical personnel to assess patient
- Early recognition and intervention for complications
- In-center treatment is safe and comfortable

Predialysis assessment of risk factors

The condition of the patient at the time dialysis is initiated plays a crucial role in survival rate. Several risk factors need to be assessed before the patient begins dialysis. These include the control of the following:
- Blood pressure
- Anemia
- Calcium/phosphorus intake
- Nutrition during the predialysis period

Comprehensive predialysis program
The areas that should be addressed in a comprehensive, multidisciplinary predialysis program include the following:
- Patient and family education
- Choice of suitable modality
- Access of dialysis
- Advantages of fewer urgent dialyses
- Fewer hospital stays in 1st month after beginning dialysis
- Significant cost savings after beginning dialysis

Membrane biocompatibility

Inflammatory responses occur when blood contacts a foreign surface. If the reaction is severe with a high level of inflammation, the membrane is bioincompatible. When the reaction is mild, the membrane is biocompatible. The complement system consists of a series of plasma proteins that react consecutively to start a series of biological occurrences. The immune system reacts to the foreign substance, the membrane, as it would to a bacterial challenge. Markers are used to evaluate the level of reaction, or the complement activation. These are C3a, C5a, which are used to describe complement activation, and C5b through C9 in the patient's blood.

Long-term use of bioincompatible and biocompatible membranes for hemodialysis

The possible negative effects of long-term usage of bioincompatible membranes are increased incidence of the following:
- Infection
- Malignancy
- Damaged nutritional state
- β2 Amyloid disease

Probable reasons for the higher incidences of these negative outcomes include the following:
- Cellulose membranes are incapable of removing large β2-Microglobulin molecules
- Due to cellulose membranes causing increased complement generation, some products of this may cause the release of $β_2$ from monocytes

Clinical manifestations that may result are as follows:
- Bone lesions
- Arthropathies
- Pathological fractures
- Soft tissue edema
- Carpal tunnel syndrome

Reaction of the body to cellulose membranes

The similarity of the cellulose surface to the cell wall of bacteria, with both being composed of polysaccharide structures, causes the body to react as if it were being attacked by bacteria. The main sources of the extreme complement activation are the free hydroxyl groups on the membrane surface. In order to diminish this reaction, chemical alterations are employed to buffer these free hydroxyl groups, producing "modified cellulosic membranes," such as cellulose acetate and Hemophan. Both modified membranes reduce the reaction, but neither is as effective as a synthetic membrane in diminishing the complement production.

Patients with some residual renal function may be negatively affected by the use of cellulose membranes. The theory postulates that the use of hemodialysis membranes that are more compatible and do not trigger complement activation leads to better recovery and survival rates. The lower the incidence of complement activation, the fewer white cells are produced and the less inflammation results. In one study, patients who were on hemodialysis with cellulose acetate membranes seemed to lose their residual renal function at a faster rate than patients who were dialyzed with a polysulfone membrane.

The practice of dialyzer reuse by the same patient after the cleaning and sterilizing of the equipment has been followed for many years. When proper techniques are used, this is a safe and cost-effective method.

Problems associated with internal AV fistulas

The most common problems associated with internal AV fistulas are as follows:
- The length of time needed for veins to be sufficiently enlarged may be an issue as this process usually takes about 6 weeks.
- Obtaining the desired blood flow may be difficult; dilation may occur in the veins on the back of the hand instead of the forearm in side-to-side anastomoses. This may require surgical correction.
- Vessel spasm causes decreased arterial flow.
- Venous stenosis or needle position may cause return-flow resistance.
- Accidental injury to the vessel during venipuncture may result in hematoma and the inability to use this site for days.
- In "radial artery steal" syndrome the radial artery has a lower arterial pressure, and the pressure gradient causes the ulnar artery blood to flow into the fistula instead of the hand and fingers, which become painful and cold. This may be surgically corrected.
- Infections are common.
- Thrombosis is the most common complication.
- Aneurysms may occur.

Black blood syndrome

A fistula with low blood flow rate may lead to recirculation. This low blood flow rate is often the result of stenosis at one of the ends of the fistula and is associated with an increase in venous pressure. Recirculation may lead to "black blood syndrome" in which the blood's acidity level increases, causing the red blood cells to lose their ability to transport oxygen. When the pH of the blood is below 7, it appears very dark in color. To test for this, 3 blood samples are taken, one from a peripheral (P) source, one from the inflow line just before it enters the dialyzer (arterial, A), and one from the outflow line just after it leaves the dialyzer (venous, V). Recirculation should remain at under 10%; if more than 15%, it is excessive and should be investigated and corrected.

Negative outcomes of using a catheter for dialysis

Venous catheters and traditional hemodialysis access sites may be used for dialysis. Patients using venous catheters may experience the following:
- A higher likelihood of infection
- Increased levels of inflammatory markers, such as C-reactive protein
- A higher mortality rate, which could be due to different patient populations, risks from receiving catheters, or some property of catheter use
- Inadequate blood flow through venous catheters
- Lower than average urea reduction rate (URR) in larger patients
- Fractional urea clearance (Kt/V) in large patients
- Lower survival rate (for catheters around 60% at 6 months and 40% at one year, if revisions are done)

Preventing hypotension

Hypotension is the most common complication seen during dialysis. Preventative measures that can be used to help avoid the complication of hypotension during dialysis are as follows:
- The ultrafiltration controller closely controls the fluid removal rate. If it is unavailable, use a membrane with low permeability to water so that transmembrane pressure fluctuations will remain small.
- Avoid interdialytic weight gain and instruct the patient to limit salt intake.
- Increase treatment time.
- Use care in determining "dry weight."
- Use correct dialysis solution sodium level.
- Maintain proper dialysate temperature.
- Avoid intradialytic food ingestion.
- Perform a predialysis test for a hemoglobin level of more than 11 g/dL (110 g/L).
- Maintain therapeutic dialysate calcium concentration (especially in cardiac patients).
- Administer antihypertensive medications after dialysis treatment, not before.

Preventing hyptensive episodes and cramping
Medications and some techniques that may be effective in the prevention of hypotensive episodes and cramping during dialysis are as follows:
- Quinine sulfate may be used to prevent cramping.
- Carnitine, oxazepam, or prazosin may reduce cramping during dialysis, although prazosin may cause hypotension.
- Stretching exercises may be beneficial in preventing cramping in certain muscles.
- Sequential compression devices may help reduce leg cramping.

The elements in the blood that need to be at appropriate levels prior to dialysis treatment are as follows:
- Magnesium
- Calcium
- Potassium

Raising the dialysis sodium level just below the level that would cause postdialysis thirst would also help with prevention of cramping.

Severe hypotension
Steps that should be taken in cases of severe hypotension that occurs during dialysis treatment are as follows:
- Place the patient in the Trendelenburg position (feet up, head down).
- Administer a bolus of 0.9% saline, 100mL or more, through the bloodline (if respiratory status tolerates).
- Reduce the ultrafiltration rate to near zero.

Muscle cramps during dialysis

Dialysis patients frequently experience muscle cramps during the first months of treatment. Factors that may contribute to muscle cramps are as follows:
- Hypotension
- Hypovolemia
- High ultrafiltration rate
- Low sodium dialysis solution
- Hypomagnesemia
- Hypocalcemia
- Hypokalemia

Reverse filtration

Reverse filtration occurs when the dialysate solution moves into the blood. This creates an unsafe condition since the water used for dialysate solution is not sterile. Bicarbonate concentrate, which may be added, promotes the growth of bacteria. Toxins and breakdown products could transfer through the membrane and into the patient's bloodstream. As a result, infections and other unfavorable reactions may develop. A molecular filter (ultrafilter) device can be used to eradicate unwanted molecular particles while allowing dissolved solutes to pass through. This filter would remove bacteria and pyrogens from the solution.

There is a possibility of reverse filtration occurring at the distal end of the dialyzer during high-flux dialysis. If reverse filtration happens during high-flux dialysis, the limulus amebocyte lysate (LAL) test is performed to determine what, if any, endotoxins are present. This test uses endotoxin units (EU) or nanograms per mL (1ng/mL=5 EU/mL). No more than 200 colony forming units (CFU) per mL of water, or 2 EU by LAL, may be present in order to meet AAMI standards.

Counter measures to ensure the safety of high-flux dialysis include the following:
- Installation of a molecular filter or ultrafilter in the dialysate line just ahead of the dialyzer may be used to filter out endotoxins
- Use of high-purity water from enhanced membrane reverse osmosis systems

Ultrafiltration profiling

The process of ultrafiltration may result in a sudden reduction of fluid in the vascular compartment. Ultrafiltration profiling refers to the ability of certain dialysis machines to fluctuate the volume of fluid removal during the treatment. The machine automatically divides the total volume to be removed (determined by the nurse) by the length of the treatment. When the ultrafiltration rate is excessive, hypovolemia and hypotension may result. In order to avoid this outcome, the use of hypertonic saline, which enhances the osmolality in the extravascular and vascular spaces, is recommended. This hypertonic solution draws fluid form the vast intracellular reservoir, avoiding the hypovolemia that leads to hypotension.

Carpal tunnel syndrome

Carpal tunnel syndrome (CTS), median neuropathy, is a compression of the median nerve at the wrist by the thickened sheath of the carpal tunnel. The cause of this thickening, in dialysis patients, is the amyloid deposition in the sheath. Carpal tunnel syndrome leads to numbness and muscle weakness in the hand, especially the thumb, index, and middle fingers. The hallmark of this syndrome is pain or numbness and tingling in these regions at night. Treatment consists of nonsteroidal anti-inflammatory drugs (NSAIDS) and ultrasound therapy. Kidney transplantation frequently leads to a prompt cessation of symptoms.

Clinical manifestations of intradialytic complement activation

The clinical manifestations of intradialytic complement activation are as follows:
- Leukopenia, a sharp drop in white cells, that corrects itself after 15 minutes and is nearly normal at the end of 4 hours, is important in patients with compromised cardiac or pulmonary function.
- C5a, the end product of the complement cascade, activates the white cells to be released and to clump, usually in the lungs.
- This reaction reduces the patient's ability to exchange O_2 and CO_2 and may result in hypoxemia.
- Symptoms of chest pain, back pain, coagulation abnormalities, and anaphylaxis may be seen.
- This reaction peaks at 15 minutes but may last up to 90 minutes.

Bicarbonate dialysate

Potential problems
Bicarbonate dialysate is an unstable solution. It requires the addition of a stabilizer, such as a polymer or dry $NaHCO_4$ powder. It is also vulnerable to bacterial contamination and once mixed the solution must be used within 24 hours. Proper sanitation of all containers and mixing apparatus is imperative to avoid contamination of the solution.

Water used for preparation
The water used for preparation of the B (bicarbonate) dialysate has to meet Advancement of Medical Instrumentation (AAMI) standards regarding the chemical make-up and pyrogen and bacterial content in order to be considered "dialysis-quality water". The microbial count has to register as less than 200 CFU/mL, and the endotoxin concentration has to be less than 2EU/mL.

Infusion of air during dialysis

When a patient receives an infusion of air during dialysis, the following steps must be taken immediately:
- Clamp the bloodlines.
- Discontinue dialysis.
- Position the patient on the left side in the Trendelenburg position (head down, feet up); this decreases air movement to the brain, traps air in the right atrium above the tricuspid valve, and diminishes foaming in right ventricle
- Maintain the airway and administer oxygen, if necessary.
- Keep the patient still and in this position for several hours for reabsorption of nitrogen and other gases.
- Obtain a chest x-ray to assess the presence of air in the heart.

Causes of chest pain

Chest pain should always be treated as cardiac in origin until proven otherwise. Dialysis patients are at increased risk for myocardial infarctions and other coronary related events. A complete history and physical must be performed with particular attention to cardiac risk factors: hypertension, diabetes mellitus, hyperlipidemia, age, history of smoking, history of stoke or heart attack, peripheral vascular disease. An electrocardiogram should be urgently done with cardiac enzymes drawn. Oxygen supplementation, morphine, nitrates, aspirin and beta blockers should also be administered. Other causes of chest pain include hemolysis, air embolism, pulmonary embolism, and hypotension.

Causes of headache, nausea and vomiting

Longer dialysis sessions and excess urea removal are frequently a root cause for headaches, nausea and vomiting. A more ominous presentation of a headache with nausea and vomiting is a myocardial infarction or early stroke. Dialysis patients are at increased risk for coronary events and this presentation may be the earliest and only signs of an impending event. Proper risk stratification with attention given to a history of hypertension, diabetes, coronary artery disease, and stroke should prompt early intervention. The dialysis disequilibrium syndrome is a rare cause of headaches. Urea removal may cause a reverse osmosis into the brain, which will cause cerebral swelling presenting as headaches and nausea. Less aggressive dialysis sessions should be curative. Other causes of headache, nausea and vomiting include caffeine withdrawal, migraine or tension headaches, metabolite disturbances (hypoglycemia, hypo and hypernatremia), medications and withdrawal from medicines.

Causes of itching

Itching is a very common complaint of dialysis patients. There are two main reasons:
- The first is an unknown complication of chronic dialysis patients.
- The second could be an indication of inadequate dialysis and thus a sign of uremia.

Frequent measuring of Kt/V would indicate the adequacy of treatments. Other causes of itching include allergies to latex and medications.

Causes of back pain

Back pain is not very specific to any particular complication but is a common complaint. Hemolysis can present as back pain as well as conditions related to the musculoskeletal system. It is also not uncommon for back pain to present as a coronary event or indigestion.

Causes of hemolysis

Hemolysis frequently presents as chest pressure, back pain and headaches. If hemolysis is suspected, urgent intervention is needed to prevent hyperkalemia. Dialysis should be immediately stopped and the root cause found. Hemolysis usually occurs with problems with the dialysis solutions. This includes:
- Overheating
- Hypotonicity
- Contamination by formaldehyde, bleach, chloramines, nitrates, and copper

The water system must be rigorously reviewed and the solutions sent for analysis of tonicity. Other causes of hemolysis include red blood cell trauma. All lines must be examined for kinks and improper clamping.

Causes of fevers and chills

Fevers and chills are frequently found in dialysis patients. The most common cause is an infection with the most common origin being the access site. Permcaths, fistulas and AV grafts are excellent sources of staphylococcus and streptococcus introductions into the blood stream. A patient with fevers, chills, hypotension or simply "toxic looking" needs two sets of blood cultures and urgent broad-spectrum antibiotics with hospitalization. Other sources of infections include viral upper respiratory infections, pneumonia, endocarditis and cellulitis. Fevers may also stem from adverse reactions to medications, allergic reactions and other inflammatory states (e.g. coronary events, gout).

Causes of arrhythmia

Arrhythmias are common in dialysis patients with the most common being ventricular arrhythmias. Treatment with varying concentrations of potassium solutions may be precipitate ventricular arrhythmias. Risk factors for arrhythmias include coronary artery disease and left ventricular cardiomyopathy. Arrhythmias are also precipitated by rapid changes in electrolyte balances during dialysis particularly potassium, calcium and magnesium. Frequent monitoring of pulse and rhythm will help the clinician identify arrhythmias early. The most dangerous rhythm is a sustained wide complex tachycardia. This is usually a ventricular tachycardia but other rhythms are possible. Wide complex tachycardia needs to be treated according to current ACLS guidelines. Supraventricular tachycardias are also common and treatment with adenosine or nodal blocking agents may be appropriate. Electroconversion is reserved for those patients with hypotension.

Disequilibrium syndrome

Disequilibrium syndrome occurs when urea is removed quickly from the patient. Urea is a major osmole in the body and its removal will cause a fluid shift from the hypoosmolar blood to the hyperosmolar cells. This is particularly concerning in brain cells and fluid shifts will cause cerebral edema and possibly brain damage. Symptoms include tremors, disorientation and convulsions. Treatment of disequilibrium includes halting dialysis and administering hypertonic saline, glucose and mannitol.

Dialyzer reaction

Dialyzer reaction occurs when the patient is first exposed to dialysis. They develop an allergic reaction and there are two forms: type A and type B.
- Type A is more severe and consists of an anaphylactoid reaction, which includes dyspnea, chest and back pain, respiratory rate increase, hypotension and possibly death. Type A reactions are usually due to exposure to ethylene oxide, a substance used in disinfecting dialyzers.
- Type B reactions are less similar but can present similarly. Treatment includes halting dialysis and administration of antihistamines.

Formaldehyde reaction

The formaldehyde reaction occurs when the patient's blood is exposed to formaldehyde. Formaldehyde is commonly used to disinfect dialyzers. When dialyzers are not properly rinsed residual formaldehyde can remain. Symptoms to formaldehyde exposure include: bitter taste, perioral numbness, chest and back pain and shortness of breath. Dialysis should be stopped.

β2 microglobulin amyloidosis in patients on dialysis

β2 microglobulin amyloidosis is a condition that is unique to patients on long-term hemodialysis and occurs rarely in patients on peritoneal dialysis. β2 microglobulin is a polypeptide that accumulates and deposits in patient's joints and tissues. Patients present with joint pain and immobility, carpal tunnel syndrome, skeletal spine immobility and gastrointestinal and heart defects. The exact etiology of the amyloidosis is unclear. The only known treatment is transplant.

Referral for evaluation when an access clot is suspected

Foremost, any abnormal finding with measurement techniques such as ultrasound or MRA should not prompt immediate evaluation. It is better to obtain serial measurements and conduct a trend analysis (with each measurement there is less flow suggesting stenosis). For AV grafts an access flow rate of less than 600 mL/min should prompt a referral. For fistulae the access flow rate should be 400- 500 mL/min. Other measurements include a venous segment static pressure ratio of greater than 0.5 in both grafts and fistulae and an arterial segment static pressure ratio greater than 0.75 in grafts. Access recirculation or inadequate dialysis (as defined by a Kt/V or Urea reduction ratio) should also lead to access evaluation. Finally and most importantly, any indication of limb ischemia at the access site requires emergent evaluation by a vascular surgeon.

Dialysis catheter dysfunction

Dialysis catheters are said to be dysfunctional or under functioning when the blood flow rate is less than 300 mL/min. Dysfunctional catheters should be treated via the following methods:
- Repositioning: Sometimes catheters can get stuck or are lodged in next to the venous wall. This will obstruct flow and repositioning the catheter will free it from adhering to the wall. Thrombolytics are indicated when there is a suspected clot in the catheter. Usually heparin is administered with each dialysis session to prevent clot formation but it is not absolute. Small thrombolytic doses can aid in breaking up a clot.
- Catheter Exchange: If the aforementioned measures fail, a catheter exchange may be needed.

Treatment for infections of AV grafts and fistulae

AV graft and fistulae infections should be treated immediately. Dialysis through infected access sites is contraindicated. The antibiotic of choice should cover both gram negative and gram-positive bacteria. Prior to antibiotics, blood cultures should be drawn. Subsequent antibiotics should be based on culture and sensitivity results. Antibiotics have to be administered intravenously to be efficacious. If the infection does not resolve, incision and drainage or complete AV graft or fistula removal may be necessary.

Treatment for infected dialysis catheters

Dialysis catheter infections are suggested when the patient presents with fever, access site induration or elevated white blood cells. The initial step is to draw two sets of blood cultures. The first should come from the dialysis catheter and the second from a peripheral site. Empiric intravenous antibiotics are indicated to cover gram-positive organisms until culture and sensitivities return. Furthermore, most dialysis catheters are in the internal jugular or subclavian veins with their tips lying near the right atrium. That leaves dialysis patients at risk for right-sided endocarditis. Thus, echocardiograms are indicated if a new regurgitant heart murmur is auscultated or with persistently positive blood cultures.

Interventions

Patient pre-assessment prior to initiation of dialysis

Areas that need to be assessed during the patient's predialysis exam include the following:
- Fluid status (heart sounds, respiration rate, effort and breath sounds, JVD, presence or absence of edema)
- Weight
- Bowel regularity
- Sleep problems
- Pain
- Residual renal function
- Bleeding or bruising
- Blood pressure, sitting and standing
- Temperature, pulse and respiration (TPR) with apical/peripheral pulse assessment
- Skin color, temperature, integrity, turgor
- Vascular access patency, lack of infection or bleeding
- Additional physical and lab data evaluation for any necessary interventions or medications needed

Physical exam findings during each dialysis session

The following physical exam findings should be noted during each dialysis session:
- Weight
- Blood pressure
- Temperature
- Pulse
- Respiratory rate
- Edema
- Assessing access site skin integrity, color and signs of inflammation
- Jugular vein distention
- Assessing access site integrity for thrills and bruits

Weighing dialysis patients

Patients are weighed before and after each dialysis session. Weight helps determine how much ultrafiltration the patient needs during dialysis. Weight is a good measure for fluid retention between dialysis sessions. Patients are advised to limit weight gain to one pound (0.5 kg) per day between dialysis. Post-dialysis weight is referred to as dry weight or the weight of the patient after fluid has been removed. Ideally, dialysis should leave the patient in a euvolemic state. Inadequate dialysis may leave patients hypervolemic and possibly hypertensive. Overadequate dialysis will leave patients hypovolemic and hypotensive.

Blood pressure measurement during dialysis

Blood pressure measurement is extremely important during dialysis. Foremost, dialysis personnel are looking for extremes of pressure (high or low). Most commonly one will encounter low blood pressures. This is usually due to the removal of fluid during dialysis. However, low blood pressures can be indicative of more serious complications including sepsis. Hypotension is a contraindication to dialysis and treatment must be stopped if the systolic blood pressure falls below 80 mm Hg. Hypertension can be an indication of hypervolemia. The high pressure can tax the heart as well as other organs. Ideally, dialysis should leave the patient in a euvolemic and normotensive state.

Monitoring nutritional status

Nutritional status is monitored through two main methods:
- The physical exam should include height, weight, weight changes, triceps skinfold and arm circumference. Serial measurements are important to trend nutritional status. The triceps skinfold and arm circumference are important indicators of body fat and protein stores.
- The biochemical tests used include albumin, prealbumin, creatinine and cholesterol. Albumin is the best studied and correlates with nutritional status and mortality. Prealbumin has a shorter half-life and can be used to monitor more acute changes. Creatinine and cholesterol are surrogate markers for protein intake and should be used to monitor nutritional status as well.

Pediatric monitoring during hemodialysis

Pediatric monitoring during dialysis includes blood pressure. This does not differ from adult monitoring. However, in children weighing less than 20 kilograms monitoring heart rate and oxygenation is required. This is done to guard against hypotension from excess fluid removal. Other signs of hypotension include lethargy, yawning and irritability. Continuous monitoring in this patient population is necessary to record subtle changes in condition.

Items necessary to conduct a predialysis machine assessment

Items necessary in dialyzer membrane check for patency and integrity:
- Blood tubing without leaks
- Accurate dialyzer
- Proper dialysate fluid composition
- Temperature limits
- Conductivity
- Extracorporeal blood circuit free of air
- Review of physician orders
- All alarms are programmed and functioning
- Dialysis water check for chloramines and other harmful agents

Parameters monitored by dialysis machine

The dialysis machine monitors the following:
- Arterial pressure
- Venous pressure
- Fluid removal
- Dialysate flow
- Blood flow
- Heparin pump
- Air leak alarm
- Blood leak alarm

Calculating transmembrane pressures for fluid removal

The transmembrane pressure can be manually entered into the dialysis machine for ultrafiltration. Today, most machines will automatically calculate the transmembrane pressure. However, knowledge of how to ascertain the transmembrane pressure is important. The formula is as follows:
- Weight to be removed in milliliters + oral fluid intake during treatment + fluid to be removed from IV infusion during treatment = total fluid to be removed.
- Total fluid to be removed/number of hours on dialysis
- Total from previous step/kuf (coefficient of dialyzer) of dialyzer = transmembrane pressure

Venous pressure

The venous pressure measures pressure in the line returning blood from the dialyzer to the patient. The venous pressure is monitored under preset parameters and alarms will sound if the pressures exceed those parameters. A sudden rise in venous pressure indicates an obstruction to flow via a clot or kink in the line. A sudden drop in venous pressure may indicate an arterial line clot or the venous needle was removed. Once activated, the alarm will halt dialysis until the problem is remedied.

Arterial pressure

The arterial pressure does not refer to the patient's systemic blood pressure. Rather, this is the pressure measured in the arterial blood line leading towards the dialysis machine. The arterial pressure is a negative pressure. That means that the blood leaving the patient is being sucked out under negative pressure as it approaches the dialysis machine. The arterial pressure is monitored with an alarm under preset ranges. A suddenly high arterial pressure is indicative of some obstruction to flow (usually a clot or kink in the line). The alarm will sound and blood flow will cease until the problem is remedied.

Appropriate history elicited from patients in preparation for access

All patients should be asked the following:
- Have you previously had a central venous catheter?
- Which is the dominant arm?
- Do you have a pacemaker?
- Do you have congestive heart failure?

- Did you recently have a large peripheral or intravenous catheter?
- Are you on anticoagulation?
- Do you have a history of valvular heart disease or valve replacement?
- Do you have a history of neck, arm or chest surgery or trauma?
- Do you have any history of failed access?

The following is a list of the clinical relevance from each of the history questions asked of patients prior to access:
- Dominant arm—Attempt to use non-dominant arm for access
- Pacemaker—Associated with central vein stenosis
- Congestive heart failure—Access can exacerbate CHF via high output cardiac failure
- Recent peripheral access—The integrity of the vein will be damaged and time is required to allow for vessel healing
- Anticoagulation—Can be a contraindication since frequent venous and arterial punctures are required
- Valvular heart disease or replacement—Access increases susceptibility of cardiac valve infections
- History of neck, arm, chest trauma/surgery—Vessel damage limits access options
- History of failed access—Limits sites where access is available

Appropriate timing and precautions to prepare patients for vascular access

Patients with chronic kidney disease stage IV and V should be made aware of their prognosis and need for renal replacement. Consent must be obtained and type of access discussed with the patient. In general, fistulas require 6 months lead time prior to dialysis, arterio-venous grafts require 3-6 weeks, peritoneal catheters need 2 weeks and permcaths can be used immediately. In preparation for permanent access, the upper extremity should not be punctured with small intravenous lines, peripheral intravenous central catheters (PICC) or subclavian catheters. This helps ensure the integrity of the native veins and arteries in preparation for fistulas and grafts.

Assessing the internal access point

The proper techniques that are recommended for assessing the internal access point before inserting the needle are as follows:
- Assess the proposed site before cleaning it.
- Observe for signs of infection: redness, inflammation, or warmth. Cold could indicate thrombosis. Check prior injection sites for healing, scabbing, and open sores. Assess for bruising, pain, numbness, or edema. If swelling is present, the circumference of the circumference should be tape-measured for later comparison to assess the progress.
- Palpate the internal access for the "thrill", a gentle vibration, which should be present over the total length. A pulse indicates less than adequate blood flow. Listen with the bell of a stethoscope for the sound of a swooshing sound, or bruit. If the bruit, swoosh and thrill are absent, the access may be clotted and should not be used.

Placement of dialysis needles

The steps used to govern the proper placement of the dialysis needles are as follows:
- The venous needle must always be placed in the same direction of the blood flow (also known as antegrade).
- The arterial needle is nearest the anastomoses (but at least 3 cm away from the site to avoid its cannulation).
- The arterial needle may be antegrade or retrograde (away from the heart).
- The venous needle must be at least 5 cm proximal to the arterial needle.
- Since the AV fistula and AV graft are cannulated at different angles, adjust insertion angle (from 20-45°) to accommodate for these differences.
- New AV fistulas are fragile and must be approached with care, usually by highly experienced personnel. It may initially be cannulated with one needle-arterial outflow, and the venous return may be accomplished by use of a central venous catheter.

Needle positioning

Needle positioning is important for many reasons. The placement of needles for dialysis should be done only after these facts are considered:
- There are potential problems with inadequate long-term patency rate of the access.
- Aneurysms may development from placing the needles in the same place, which affects vessel walls by making them become thin.
- Needle sites must be rotated to avoid this weakening of vessel walls.
- Placing the arterial needle near the anastomoses achieves optimal blood flow.
- The needle tip should remain more than 3 cm away from anastomoses.
- The usual practice is to place the arterial needle with the flow.
- Spacing needles 5cm apart minimizes recirculation of the blood, which could lead to inadequate dialysis.

Buttonhole technique of accessing a vascular access point

The buttonhole technique is a constant site technique in which an AV fistula is accessed for cannulation through the exact same site and at the same angle, creating a tunnel tract of scar tissue. This tract allows for easier cannulation, using the same scarred channel each time. This results in less pain for the patient and fewer cases of infiltration and may be a helpful alternative for the patient who dialyzes at home. Medisystems has a dull needle for use once the buttonhole is fully developed; this prevents the patient from cutting the tissue encircling the tunnel track.

Preferred access types

According to the National Kidney Foundation, access types should be in the following order of preference:
- Fistulae are preferred in the following order:
    1. Wrist (radiocephalic) primary fistula
    2. Elbow (brachiocephalic) primary fistula
    3. Transposed brachial basilic vein

- Arterio-venous grafts are less preferred than fistulae. They should be placed at the following locations in descending order:
    1. Forearm
    2. Upper arm
    3. Chest wall or lower extremity
- Long-term catheters should be generally avoided. In order of descending preference:
    1. Long term (tunnel cuffed) catheters
    2. Short term catheters

AV graft

Arteriovenous grafts are a conduit between arteries and veins. A synthetic (most common) or biocompatible conduit is inserted subcutaneously connecting an artery with a vein. Blood flows from the artery into the graft and empties in the vein. The graft requires 2-6 weeks to mature. It is important to note the direction of blood flow. Blood returning from the hemodialysis machine must enter the venous line and flow in the same direction as arterial blood. This will ensure that venous resistance is not high and that physiologic flow in the body is maintained without too much turbulence. It will also help prevent recirculation (already dialyzed blood returning to the dialyzer).

Advantages of arterio-venous grafts

AV grafts have the following advantages:
- Large vessel for easier access during dialysis
- Shorter time to maturation for use (3-6 weeks)
- Many insertion sites
- Technically easier for surgeons
- Easy to repair

Normal physical findings for AV grafts

The normal physical findings for AV grafts include:
- No irregular areas or sites of aneurysms
- Low pitch systolic and diastolic sounds
- Thrill palpated best at the arterial anastomosis but also throughout the graft with easy compressibility

Arteriovenous fistula

Fistulae are created by vascular surgeons. Small incisions are made in the forearm or elbow and an adjoining artery and vein is anastomosed. The increased blood flow from the artery into the vein causes venous dilation. The vein must be allowed to fully dilate and mature which is about a six-month process. Fistulae are the most preferred method for hemodialysis access because of their decreased infection and clotting rates. The procedure is usually done in an office setting and is relatively quick. Arm exercises are also prescribed to the patient to help facilitate fistula maturation.

Normal physical findings for AV fistulae

The normal physical findings for fistulae include:
- Well developed venous outflow with no areas of aneurysms
- The vessels partially collapse when the patient raises his/her arm above head
- Low pitch diastolic and systolic murmur with auscultation
- Thrill felt best at the arterial site but can be felt throughout the entire outflow vein

Needles used for puncturing the AV fistula

The preferred type of needle that is used to accommodate high blood flows in high-flux or high-efficiency dialyzers have the following features:
- The preferred needle type has a large gauge, which allows for high blood flows, high-flux, or high-efficiency dialysis. Blood flows of 400-500 mL/min with 14-gauge needles, 17- gauge are used in children and infants, although it is recommended to use at least a 15-gauge, which accommodates a large volume of blood flow of 350 mL/min or more. Dialyzing with a small gauge needle may cause hemolysis of red-blood cells due to the cells passing through the needle with such force that they are ruptured.
- The preferred needle type has a thin-wall.
- The preferred needle type has a back-eye.

Advantages of fistulae over other access types

Fistulae are recommended by the National Kidney Foundation because of their lower complication rates. Foremost, they have the lowest rate of thrombosis and failures. Thus, they require fewer interventions, which make them very cost effective. Fistulae do not get infected as often as permcaths or grafts. The combination of the stated advantages leads to lower hospitalizations and increased survival for dialysis patients.

Wrist and elbow fistulae

The wrist and elbow offer the following advantages:
- Greater patency to flow after maturing
- Lower rates of stenosis, infection and vascular steal (the new conduit "steals" blood from the radial artery).

The disadvantages include:
- Long time to mature (usually 1 – 4 months)
- Difficulty accessing the vein during dialysis relative to grafts
- Cosmetically displeasing

The wrist is the first choice by surgeons in choosing access sites. The reasons include:
- Technically easy site to work with
- Preserves proximal vessels in case the fistula fails
- Fewer adverse events including thrombosis, infections and vascular steal.

The major disadvantage to wrist fistulae is that it offers a lower blood flow rate in comparison to more proximal, larger vessels. The elbow is the second choice for fistulae behind the wrist.

The major advantages include:
- Higher blood flow rate
- Easier to cannulate for hemodialysis access (large vessel)

The disadvantages include:
- Technically more difficult for surgeons
- More edema
- Higher incidence of vascular steal and stenosis

Cannulating a mature fistula or graft

The following is the proper technique for cannulating a mature fistula or graft:
- First, the skin is prepped with proper infection control techniques.
- A tourniquet must be applied proximal to the fistula. This will decrease venous return and help engorge the fistula for easier access.
- Then pull the skin in the opposite direction from needle insertion.
- For arterial puncture, the needle can be either in the same or opposite direction as blood flow.
- For venous punctures, the needle must be inserted in the same direction as blood flow.
- After inserting the needle it should be advanced slowly and taped to the skin surface.
- Once dialysis is over the needle should be removed at the same angle as it was inserted (this prevents vessel tearing).
- Pressure should not be applied to the needle site until after it is removed (to avoid vessel trauma and blood splashes).

Fistula and graft surveillance of patency

It is important to monitor patency of both fistulae and grafts to ensure adequate dialysis and continued access. The National Kidney Foundation lists the following techniques as preferred or acceptable means of monitoring access patency:
- Doppler ultrasound
- Magnetic resonance angiography (MRA)
- Various dilution techniques
- Physical findings

The physical findings include loss of palpable thrill, lack of bruit on auscultation, persistent arm swelling, presence of collateral veins and prolonged bleeding.

Monitoring, surveillance and diagnostic testing as related to vascular access

Monitoring refers to the examination and evaluation of the vascular access via physical examination to detect physical signs that suggest the presence of dysfunction. Surveillance is the periodic evaluation of the vascular access by using tests that may involve special instrumentation and for which an abnormal test result suggests the presence of dysfunction. Diagnostic testing refers to specialized testing that is prompted by some abnormality or other medical indication and that is undertaken to diagnose the cause of the vascular access dysfunction.

Preference of fistulae and grafts over long-term catheters

Long-term catheters (permcaths) are associated with high infection rates and are frequently clotted. Furthermore, a permcath placed in the subclavian or internal jugular veins drains near the right atrium. This will subject the patient's cardiac valves (particularly tricuspid) to infections by staphylococcus and streptococcus. Fistulae and grafts also last longer, decrease hospitalizations, and improve patients' quality of life. All long-term catheters should be placed with plans for more permanent access.

Dialysis catheter

The use of the central venous catheter may result in subclavian vein stenosis; therefore, it should only be chosen as a temporary alternative to traditional modes of hemodialysis. The situations that would indicate the use of a dialysis catheter in a hemodialysis patient are as follows:
- When the need arises for acute dialysis access, before mature access
- For the patient with an imminent kidney transplantation surgery
- When awaiting the AV access maturation
- When the availability of appropriate vessels is limited for permanent internal access
- For the patient receiving plasmapheresis
- For patient receiving venovenous continuous renal replacement therapy
- For patient with peritonitis who usually use peritoneal dialyses
- For patients who have acute overdose or intoxication

Catheter types

Different types of catheters used for dialysis include the following:
- Cuffed and uncuffed: Uncuffed catheters when used over a prolonged period are often associated with a high infection rate. Cuffed are preferable due to their Dacron or felt cuffs, which reduce the incidence of infection and catheter migration.
- Dual-lumen catheters in a side-by-side (double-D) configuration result in less recirculation and have a larger separation of inlet and outlet ports and more pliable catheters.
- The palindrome symmetrical tip reduces recirculation.
- The Tesio catheter system features 2 separate catheters, one for inflow and one for outflow, made of softer silicone material.

Veins chosen for temporary vascular access

Veins chosen for temporary vascular access are the subclavian, internal jugular, and femoral veins. Subclavian and jugular veins are used in certain patients, but for others these sites are contraindicated.
- Patients with difficulty breathing who cannot be placed in supine or Trendelenburg positions, and those with subclavian vein stenosis are not candidates for subclavian or jugular access.
- The right internal jugular is the optimal insertion site. The subclavian vein should not be used due to the complications that may result, including hemothorax, pneumothorax, subclavian artery perforation, brachial plexus injury, and a higher rate of venous stenosis. For short-term catheter placement, the femoral artery is a good choice. If a femoral catheter is used, it should be at least 20cm in length to assure that the tip is located in the inferior vena cava for good blood flow and to minimize recirculation.

Femoral catheter

There are certain times that the use of a femoral catheter for dialysis is indicated. These are as follows:
- When an acutely ill patient is confined to bed
- When dialysis is needed immediately and the access is compromised as in the end stage renal disease (ESRD) patient
- For continuous renal replacement treatment
- When the patient has subclavian vein stenosis

Complications that may occur immediately after insertion of a catheter into the femoral vein are as follows:
- Pneumothorax
- Hemothorax
- Air embolism
- Bleeding from inadvertent puncture of femoral artery

Infection at catheter site

One of the complications of catheter placement that may occur is infection. Signs and symptoms of infection at the catheter site include the following:
- Fever or chills
- Severe cases exhibit hemodynamic instability
- Septic symptoms

Causative agents are frequently Gram-positive organisms, usually of the Staphylococcus species, but Gram-negative may be associated with up to 40% of infections. Treatment begins with blood cultures and continues with administration of systemic antibiotics that cover both Gram-positive and Gram-negative bacteria. Vancomycin should be given a methicillin-resistant Staphylococcus has been detected in the dialysis population. Removal of the catheter is recommended. One week after the completion of antibiotic therapy, blood cultures should be repeated.

Limitations of placing long-term catheters

Permcaths should not be placed in the following two regions:
- Where current or future AV access is maturing or to be placed
- In femoral veins in patients waiting for transplants.

Arterio-venous fistulae need time to mature as do AV grafts. Thus, placing a permcath near the site of maturing or future access sites will endanger the fistula or graft. In patients on the transplant list, access via the femoral vein should be avoided. The reasoning includes placing the patient at risk for femoral vein thrombosis. The femoral vein is near the renal vein and anything that may compromise that vasculature should be avoided.

Tunneled cuffed catheters

Tunneled cuffed catheters offer the following advantages:
- All patients can receive them
- Easily inserted at various sites
- Can be used immediately post insertion
- Skin puncture is not necessary
- No hemodynamic consequences, e.g. high output cardiac failure
- Low costs
- Can be used as short term brides until grafts and fistulae mature

The major disadvantages of tunneled catheters include:
- High rates of infection
- High rates of thrombosis
- Central venous stenosis
- Cosmetically displeasing
- Short shelf life
- Lower blood flow rates which increases dialysis times

LifeSite Hemodialysis Access System

The LifeSite Hemodialysis Access System refers to an implantable device that is used as a central venous blood access port for hemodialysis. The system is comprised of a 1.2-inch round, 0.5-inch high metal valve with a 25-inch cannula line. The valve is placed subcutaneously with the cannula extending into the subclavian or jugular vein. Two systems are placed in the patient for both the draw and return of blood. A specialized 14 gauge needle is inserted into the LifeSite valve; this opens the internal pinch clamp, allowing for the flow of blood. Removing the needle allows the clamp to close. After several cannulations into the valve, a tract or buttonhole is created between the skin and valve entrance. An antimicrobial solution is used to irrigate the pocket valve between treatments.

Contraindications and possible complications
Contraindications associated with using the LifeSite Hemodialysis Access System include the following:
- Positive blood cultures associated with recent infection
- Systemic or localized infection that does not respond to antibiotic therapy
- Lack of adequate tissue to support placement of the valve
- Confirmed or suspected allergy to components of the device

Possible complications of the LifeSite Hemodialysis Access System are as follows:
- Inadequate blood flow
- Bleeding or hematoma at injection site
- Cannulation problems
- Thrombosis
- Site infections
- Valve pocket or cannula tunnel infections
- Bacteremia or septicemia

Monitoring hemoglobin levels

The best time to draw hemoglobin and hematocrit levels is predialysis. While one could argue that a post-dialysis measurement of hemoglobin would be more accurate because is approximates the patient's dry weight, most studies have only examined predialysis levels. Moreover, all of the guidelines for management of anemia in patients on hemodialysis are based on predialysis data. Therefore, it is accepted practice and by convention that one draws and interprets the predialysis hemoglobin/hematocrit.

Urea reduction ratio

The urea reduction ratio is the percentage of urea removed during dialysis. The postdialysis urea is subtracted from the predialysis urea to give the amount that was removed. This amount is then divided by the predialysis urea and multiplied by 100% to give the percentage removed:
$$(BUN_{pre} - BUN_{post})/BUN_{pre} \times 100\%$$

An adequate urea reduction ratio is 65%. The urea reduction ratio is another indicator of dialysis adequacy.

Drawing predialysis BUN from patients with AV fistulas, grafts, and permcaths

In patients with AV fistulas or grafts, the predialysis BUN should be drawn prior to initiating hemodialysis. The sample should be taken from the arterial port. The syringe should be free of any saline or heparin so as not to dilute the sample. In patients with permcaths, the first 5 cc of blood should be drawn and discarded. This ensures that any remaining heparin or saline that remains in the catheter is discarded. Than the sample should be drawn and sent for analysis. Again, this should be done prior to the initiation of hemodialysis. The blood sample needs to be drawn under sterile technique.

Collecting post dialysis BUN samples

Post dialysis BUN samples should be collected as follows:
- First, the dialysate flow should be stopped or decreased to the lowest permitted setting for 3 minutes.
- Then the blood flow rate should be decreased to 100 mL/min for 15 seconds. This prevents auto recirculation of blood from artificially diluting the BUN and falsely elevating Kt/V.
- After the 15 seconds, the blood pump should be stopped and the sample can be drawn under sterile technique. Blood should be obtained from either the arterial port side.

Again, waiting 15 seconds under the low flow rate is important to obtain an accurate post BUN sample.

Dialysis adequacy

Dialysis adequacy is measured with the formula Kt/V. Kt/V is a complex formula that assesses how well each dialysis session went. The K represents a kinetic factor for urea, t is for dialysis time and v is a calculated guess at the volume of distribution for urea. Memorizing the exact calculations involved is not necessary but a pre- and post-dialysis BUN is required along with pre- and post-dialysis weights. The former is an indication of urea clearance and the latter for volume removed. Current guidelines suggest a Kt/V of greater than 1.2. A level of less than 1.2 indicates inadequate dialysis and is associated with worse outcomes. All dialysis centers keep track of Kt/V for all patients as a metric of quality control.

According to the National Kidney Foundation, dialysis adequacy can be adversely affected via three main categories:
1. compromised urea clearance
2. reduced treatment time
3. laboratory errors

Urea clearance can be compromised through the following:
- Access recirculation
- Inadequate blood flow from vascular access
- Inaccurate estimation of dialyzer performance
- Inadequate dialyzer reprocessing
- Clotted dialyzer fibers
- Errors in blood and dialysate flow rates caused by miscalibrated equipment
- Inadequate blood and dialysate flow rate
- Dialyzer leaks

Reduced treatment time can occur with early discontinuation of treatment, inaccurate time of dialysis recorded and not accounting for interruptions during dialysis treatments. Finally, laboratory errors occur with dilution of BUN blood samples, drawing pre and post dialysis BUN at the wrong time, laboratory errors and drawing post dialysis BUN after more than five minutes after the end of dialysis.

Education

Predialysis education

The most important predialysis education goals include these:
- Supply information about preferred dialysis modalities
- Endorse home dialysis
- Encourage responsibility and self-reliance for personal health

When GFR is 20mL/min or the condition is rapidly declining, these procedures should be followed:
- Use written materials
- Encourage internet research
- Suggest group sessions
- Provide individual sessions with dialysis nurse

Group sessions should do the following:
- Allow time for patients to interact with others with similar health concerns
- Encourage discussion of dialysis modalities
- Invite current dialysis patients for personal insights

Individual sessions should follow these guidelines:
- Be scheduled after group sessions
- Respond to questions arising from group discussions
- Assess patient's comprehension of dialysis treatment alternatives
- Incorporate a visit to PD and HD training facilities and interactions with patients currently in training

Critical signs and symptoms to be aware of post-dialysis

Electrolyte abnormalities can develop following dialysis, with hyperkalemia being the most common. Symptoms the patient may experience with this include numbness or tingling and palpitations, though it is usually asymptomatic. Other electrolyte abnormalities that can occur include hyponatremia, hypocalcemia, and hypermagnesemia. Dialysis disequilibrium syndrome is common and is characterized by weakness, dizziness, and headache. Mental status changes can occur in severe cases. The patient should monitor their fistula site for any acute signs of infection. It should also be palpated for a thrill. The absence of a thrill may indicate a blood clot. Bleeding from a vascular access site may occur due to the heparin often used in dialysis to prevent clotting. This can usually be controlled with elevation and pressure at the site. Patients receiving peritoneal dialysis need to be alert for the signs of peritonitis, which include abdominal pain or a cloudy effluent. Peritonitis occurs approximately once per patient per year. Patients should also be aware of the common symptoms of anemia because this is common with kidney failure.

Renal replacement therapy modalities

The patient needs to be made aware of all of the options available for the treatment of renal replacement therapy. These include the following:
- Pre-emptive kidney transplantation: survival superior to standard dialysis
- Dialysis, home vs. in-center therapy: availability in local area, transportation issues, status of patient's home, support structure, technical issues
- Short daily hemodialysis, 5 day a week treatments decrease cramping and hypotension
- Long nocturnal dialysis, 8-10 hours in length, usually done at home
- Peritoneal dialysis, decreases requirement for special water systems, simple equipment setup, better mobility
- Palliative care with no dialysis

Methods of monitoring nutritional status

Other than serum laboratory tests and physical exams, methods of monitoring nutritional status include the following:
- Taking dietary history and keeping diaries
- Use of the subjective global assessment survey (a validated survey looking at patient's total well being)
- Protein catabolic rate (examines the difference between nitrogen intake and waste)
- Dual Energy X-ray Absorptiometry (DEXA) scans (whole body DEXA scans are a reliable way to examine body composition irrespective of fluid status)

Dietary restrictions in patients with chronic kidney disease stages II-IV

Patients with chronic kidney disease should adopt the following dietary habits:
- Low protein
- Low sodium
- Low phosphorus

The low protein diet is helpful in reducing the amount of nitrogenous waste produced with protein breakdown. Nitrogenous wastes help contribute towards uremia. A low phosphorus diet is also important to limit the amount of phosphorus absorption. Increased phosphorus coupled with calcium can lead to calcium-phosphate deposition into tissues causing damage and ischemia. Finally, limiting sodium intake is crucial to lowering blood pressure and decrease water retention. Hypertension is both a cause and a consequence of renal failure and sodium restriction has been implicated in causing and exacerbating high blood pressure.

Dietary restrictions on potassium and phosphorus in patients on dialysis

Potassium should be limited to approximately 70 mEq/day. Multiple factors are involved in regulating potassium intake including size of the patient, dialysate used and medications. An excellent source (hazard) of potassium includes vegetables and fruits, particularly bananas. Phosphorus intake should be limited to 600 – 1200 mg/day. Phosphorus intake is largely controlled by phosphate binders and an excellent source of phosphorus includes protein and soda.

Protein intake requirements

Patients on hemodialysis should aim for a goal of 1.2 gm/kg of body weight per day. Patients on peritoneal dialysis should aim for a goal of 1.3 gm/kg of body weight per day. Patients on dialysis have higher protein requirements because they lose amino acids with each dialysis session. Moreover, malnutrition is a problem with dialysis patients and studies have shown that low albumin is correlated with increased hospitalizations. Proteins come from two sources: animal and plant.
- Animal sources include all essential amino acids and good choices include fish, chicken.
- Plant sources include legumes and nuts.

Water intake

Water intake is largely contingent on urine formation plus insensible losses. The ability to closely match water intake with output will help with water homeostasis and maintain balance. Thus, water input is entirely patient specific. If, however, the patient does not make any urine than only insensible losses should be recovered. Excess water intake leads to hypertension exacerbation and left ventricular hypertrophy. Acceptable limits to weight gain between dialysis sessions is 1.5 kg.

Vitamin supplementation and trace minerals

Vitamin supplementation may be necessary in patients on dialysis. Dialysis patients are at risk for vitamin deficiencies, particularly water-soluble vitamins. Supplementation with vitamins B1, B2, B6, B12 and niacin and folate is acceptable. Excess vitamins A and C should be avoided for they are toxic in renal patients. Trace minerals do not need to be replaced routinely. A daily multivitamin is more than enough to replace the needed minerals lost.

Providing supplemental nutrition

There are essentially three ways of supplying supplemental nutrition:
- Orally
- Intradialytic parenteral nutrition
- Intraperitoneal amino acid dialysate for peritoneal dialysis patients

Oral supplementation usually comes as protein shakes such as Ensure. Intradialytic parenteral nutrition (IDPN) is the administration of proteins and calories during dialysis. It is used in patients who cannot take or do not adequately respond to oral supplements. For peritoneal dialysis patients, intraperitoneal amino acid dialysate is used. Amino acids are substituted for a portion of the dextrose and have been shown to increase protein intake.

Dietary differences between peritoneal dialysis and hemodialysis patients

Peritoneal dialysis patients require some differences in dietary intake. Foremost, they require more protein due to the larger protein losses with peritoneal dialysis. The caloric intake is similar for both patients but the peritoneal patient absorbs more dextrose. The dextrose adds more calories and can exacerbate hypertriglyceridemia in obese diabetics or be helpful in undernourished patients. Sodium and fluid intake not need be as stringent as with hemodialysis patients. This is due to the ability of the dialysate to remove excess fluid with more frequent exchanges. Potassium is also less of a problem because of the infusion of insulin with each exchange. The insulin forces potassium into the cells and lowers serum K levels. However, phosphorus is more difficult to control in peritoneal dialysis patients. The phosphorus is usually accompanied with protein and thus more phosphate binders are required.

Medication Administration

Volume of distribution

Volume of distribution refers to the volume of plasma required to maintain a certain concentration of a drug. It is defined by the equation:
> Volume of distribution = Total amount of drug in the body/drug concentration.

The volume of distribution is not a real volume but an arbitrary value. Drugs that are absorbed into the blood are either protein bound or free. Because nly the free drug is active, a highly bound drug is said to have a small volume of distribution. In dialysis, increased fluid retention coupled with lower albumin (malnutrition) leads to increased volume of distribution. In addition, the increased serum acidity alters how albumin binds to medications, which often leads to a more free drug. Thus, most drugs need to be given at lower doses or with less frequency.

Bioavailability

Bioavailability refers to the amount of drug that is absorbed and becomes available for use. Bioavailability is largely contingent on route of administration, intrinsic characteristics of the drug and environmental factors. Drugs can be administered orally, subcutaneously, intramuscularly or intravenously, or can be inhaled. Each route will offer a different bioavailability. For example, an oral drug has to get absorbed from the gut and pass through the liver before being available for use while an intravenous medication is not subject to the gut or liver. Thus, for a given drug dosage the bioavailability of an intravenous administration is higher than oral. In dialysis patients, uremia alters the stomach pH (higher than normal). The lower acidity alters drug absorption. Other medications taken such as phosphate binders and H2 blockers also alter gut pH. Finally, uremia alters liver enzymatic activity. Some drugs are more available whereas others are less so.

Half-life

Half-life is the amount of time needed for the body to eliminate 50% of a drug. This is an exponential decline in drug concentration and half-life is useful in helping one deduce how long a drug will remain active in the body. In dialysis patients, the half-life of medicines is increased. This is secondary to larger volumes of distribution and lower clearance rates.

Clearance

Clearance can be understood by the simple equation:
$$\text{clearance} = \text{rate of drug removal/concentration}.$$

Clearance is the volume of blood that is completely removed from a substance over time. However, clearance is not simply clearing the blood of a drug or toxin but rather how that substance is removed from the blood. For example, both urea and glucose are filtered at the glomerulus. Urea is cleared by the kidney at a rate of 65mL/min. In contrast, glucose is cleared by the kidney at 0 mL/min. That means that glucose is filtered by the kidney but is completely reabsorbed and thus its clearance is zero. Urea, on the other hand, is not completely reabsorbed and so its clearance is higher. In dialysis patients, the clearance for most drugs is lower. This is because not all drugs are dialyzable (only small molecular weight medicines are dialyzed). Clearance is useful in monitoring maintenance doses and in dialysis patients the doses are usually decreased.

Medications for ESRD patients

Selection of a medication to treat an ESRD patient requires special consideration by the physician. The effects on kidney function, electrolyte balance, and uremia must be taken into account. Any agent that will cause an increase in the metabolite load or be a detriment to the disease state should be avoided. Any drug that increases levels of urea, sodium, potassium, or acids further stresses the already failing kidney. Nephrotoxic drugs should also be used with great care. If possible, a single drug that can treat multiple conditions is preferable over numerous agents.

Loading dose and maintenance dose

"Loading dose" refers to the amount or dosage of a drug that must be administered in order to obtain a therapeutic plasma level as quickly as possible. Loading doses can be dangerous because of their rapid administration technique and the increase in the blood plasma level of the drug. Loading doses are found in the drug reference literature but are calculated as the product of the required plasma concentration level (blood level "Cp") and the volume of distribution of the medication. The formula is as follows:
$$\text{Loading dose (mg/kg)} = V_d \text{ (mL/kg)} \times C_p \text{ (mg/mL)}$$

Once this value is determined in mg/kg, multiply this dose by the patient's ideal weight.

Need for anticoagulation during dialysis

When blood comes into contact with dialyzers and tubing it tends to clot. The dialyzer and tubing are foreign substances that aid in clot formation. Moreover, access sites have a high tendency to clot. The order of clot formation in descending order is: catheter>graft>fistula. In order to prevent clots in either access or extracorporeal sites, anticoagulation is administered. The most commonly used anticoagulant is heparin. Heparin is well tolerated in dialysis patients because of its relatively short half-life. Also, should bleeding ensue an antidote is readily available to reverse heparin's affects (protamine sulfate).

Anticoagulation in pediatric hemodialysis

Anticoagulation in pediatrics is similar to that of adults. The heparin dose is weight based and thus both loading and maintenance doses are adjusted to the child's weight. The same goals of therapy hold. The activated clotting time should be approximately 1.5 times normal. However, neonates and children with little mass need tight controls of the adjusted clotting times. This particular population is subject to cerebral hemorrhage from heparin.

Regional heparinization

Regional heparinization refers to the continual infusion of heparin via the arterial line with a concurrent infusion of an antidote into the venous line before the blood is infused back into the patient. Trisodium citrate is used in the arterial line. Since a calcium-free dialysate must be used with trisodium citrate, calcium chloride must be added into the venous line to prevent blood returning to the patient with a low ionized calcium level. The major disadvantages of this type of heparinization are that numerous laboratory tests are required to assess the clotting time and calcium levels.

Tight heparinization

"Tight heparinization" which is also known to as low-dose heparinization, refers to the technique of heparin administration in which the dosage is determined by frequent clotting times in order to maintain a clotting time of 90-120 seconds by ACT. This technique is often used for the patient's first dialysis treatment or for any patient at risk for bleeding, such as one who is menstruating, post surgery, or who has a central venous catheter that will be removed postdialysis. After the minimal priming dose is given, the usual dosage is 10 units/kg and is regulated to maintain an ACT of 110 ± 10 seconds.

Administration of heparin for dialysis patients

Assuming the patient is not a risk for bleeding, there are two main methods of heparin administration. The first is called intermittent intravenous heparin technique. It involves a loading dose at the beginning of dialysis with intermittent, smaller doses later on. The goal of treatment is to keep the clotting time between 150 – 180 seconds (three times normal). The second technique is called continuous infusion which involves a loading dose of heparin given systemically. Heparin is than slowly given to the extracorporeal system only throughout dialysis. Clotting times are used to adjust heparin infusions.

Risks and safe administration

Heparin is an anticoagulant and thus places the patient at increased risk of bleeding. Patients who are at increased risk of bleeding should not receive heparin during dialysis. These include:
- Patients who are actively bleeding
- Have a clotting disorder
- Take anticoagulants
- Recent surgery
- Recent trauma
- Thrombocytopenia
- Allergic to heparin

Patients at increased bleeding risk should not receive heparin at all. Furthermore, dialysis patients have poorly functioning platelets and thus cannot easily form a clot to prevent bleeding. In order to safely administer heparin the following should be done:
- Base the heparin dose on the patient's dry weight
- Check clotting times every 30 minutes
- Check the dialyzer and tubing for evidence of clots
- Check the patient for evidence of ecchymosis
- Stop heparin 30 – 60 minutes before the completion of dialysis

Hemodialysis done without heparinization

Hemodialysis done without the use of an anticoagulant is the therapy of choice for patients with an increased risk of bleeding, pericarditis, coagulopathy, or thrombocytopenia. The most common methods used are as follows:
- Bloodlines and dialyzer are primed with saline with 3000 units of heparin/L, and then this solution is discarded (this technique is not used for patients with extremely high risk of bleeding, such as liver disease).
- Blood flow rates are set as high as tolerated, 350-450 mL/min.
- The dialyzer is rinsed with 100-200 mL of saline as frequently as every 15 minutes up to once every hour, through the arterial line, and is inspected for clotting.

Reversing drug-induced renal damage

Drug-induced renal damage can often be reversed and further damage prevented if the following steps are taken:
- Discontinue nephrotoxic drug immediately.
- Administer saline intravenously to decrease nephrotoxins such as cyclosporine or cisplatin by dilution of the drugs in the renal tubules.
- Damage done by nonsteroidal anti-inflammatory agents (NSAIDS) may be diminished by administering misoprostol, a prostaglandin analog.
- Select drugs with the least probability of nephrotoxicity, such as acetaminophen, aspirin, nonacetylated salicylates, sulindac, or nabumetone.
- Give lowest effective dose of any drug for the shortest duration for effectiveness.

Psychological and Sociocultural Interventions

Psychological reactions in coping with dialysis

The most common reactions include:
- Anxiety—The most common initial reaction. Patients and their families are about to embark on a very new experience and significant life style changes are about to take place. Dialysis staff needs to be supportive.
- Depression—On the same spectrum as anxiety and the two emotions often coincide. Again, the uncertainty of life on dialysis along with life style changes leads to these feelings.
- Anger—Can be manifested in many ways. Often dialysis patients are frustrated with their disease but will express anger towards their family or staff.

In all three instances referral to a social worker or psychiatrist is important in helping patients and families cope.

Psychological stages of adjustment after beginning dialysis

There are three stages of psychological adjustment once dialysis is started:
1. Honeymoon Period—When a patient first undergoes dialysis. This period usually lasts from 6 weeks to 6 months. The patient feels better about their prognosis and carries a positive outlook.
2. Period of Disenchantment and Discouragement—Patients experience a loss of hope and confidence. As they settle into life on dialysis they begin to realize the restrictions it has on their lifestyle.
3. Period of Long-Term Adaptation—The patient begins to accept life with dialysis and all that it carries. Patients settle in to a routine with intermittent periods of depression.

Stressors experienced by ESRD patients

Dialysis patients often experience a variety of psychosocial stressors due to their chronic illness and time-consuming treatments. Some of the physical, psychological and psychiatric problem areas may include the following:
- Effects of the illness
- Dietary restrictions
- Scheduling constraints
- Fear of dying
- Marital discord, sexual dysfunction, hormonal effects
- Tense interpersonal relationships with family, medical staff, administrative personnel
- Expense of treatment
- Unemployment
- Psychological complaints, anxiety, anger, hostility and depression with feelings of lack of worth, lack of interest in daily activities, changes in weight, altered sleep patterns, fatigue, inability to concentrate and thoughts of suicide
- Psychiatric disorders such as dementia, delirium, psychosis, anxiety disorders, and drug abuse

Depression in the ESRD patient

Treatment for depression in the dialysis patient may include drug therapy such as the following:
- Selective serotonin reuptake inhibitors (SSRIs) and tricyclic antidepressants (TCAs) must be taken for 4-6 weeks to see the effects.
- Selective norepinephrine reuptake inhibitors (SNRIs) must be used with caution in dialysis patients since they are excreted through the kidneys.
- Monoamine oxidase inhibitors (MAOIs) should be avoided due to potential for causing hypotension.

Nonpharmacologic options include the following:
- Psychotherapy (cognitive, behavioral, interpersonal, and supportive), group therapy or individual
- Electroconvulsive therapy, if no contraindications

Infection Control

Hand washing

Studies have shown that dirty hands are the number one reason for infections traveling from patient to patient, patient to staff, or staff to patient. Frequent hand washing with soap and water or with an alcohol based cleanser is required. Moreover, anytime a health care provider travels from patient to patient, they should wash their hands.

Standard precautions implemented in dialysis units

Standard precautions include the following:
- Barrier precautions which includes gloves, face shield masks and gowns
- Protection against sharps and needles (sharps container)
- Personal hygiene (hand washing)
- Avoidance of environmental contamination (no eating, drinking, smoking in the treatment room)

Barrier precautions in dialysis centers

The most commonly used barrier precautions include:
- Gloves
- Face shield masks
- Gowns

They are used to protect both patient and nurse from transmitted blood borne as well as other infectious agents. Gloves are to be worn whenever contacting blood, bodily fluids, mucous membranes or soiled products. Between patients, hand washing and glove changes are necessary. Face shield masks are used during any procedure when there is a risk of a blood splash. This includes cannulation of an AV graft or fistula as well as decannulation at the end of dialysis. Gowns should be worn to protect the body against blood splashes or bodily fluids coming in contact with the health care provider.

Common blood borne pathogens

The most common blood borne pathogens include:
- Hepatitis B
- Hepatitis C
- HIV, Hepatitis D
- Cytomegalovirus

The most commonly transmitted virus is Hepatitis B. All healthcare workers as well as dialysis patients should be immunized against Hepatitis B. Furthermore, immunization against Hepatitis B renders immunity against Hepatitis D. HIV transmission is also concerning but is not as easily transferable as Hepatitis B. In fact, the risk of acquiring HIV from a known HIV patient from a needle stick is 0.3%. Currently there is no vaccine against Hepatitis C. Cytomegalovirus is readily found in most people and is only an issue in the immunocompromised e.g. persons with HIV or on immunosuppressive therapy.

Prophylaxis in staff after accidental needle stick

In the event of a needle stick the most important thing is to thoroughly cleanse the wound. A thorough history from the patient is necessary. The main concern is for blood borne pathogens, specifically Hepatitis B, Hepatitis C and HIV. The following table describes what actions to take:
- Suspect Hepatitis B: If staff member is immune, check immune status. If staff member is unsure of immunity, check immune status and if okay than no further treatment. If staff member is not immune, give Anti-HB immunoglobulin and initiate vaccination.
- Suspect Hepatitis C: Check Hepatitis C viral RNA, anti-HCV antibodies and liver function tests at baseline and 4-6 weeks and 4-6 months. There is no current recommendation for prophylaxis.
- Suspect HIV: Give two or three drugs post exposure for prophylaxis treatment depending on risk factors of the source. Baseline, 6 weeks, 12 weeks and 6 months testing for HIV should be done.
- Patients are asked to get tested for the aforementioned viruses if they are unsure of their status. However, they are not obligated to consent for any of these tests.

Hepatitis B

Transmission
Hepatitis B is a DNA virus transmitted through the blood. It is commonly transmitted through needles, perinatally, sexually, nosocomially (in hospital and outpatient care facilities), or via transfusions and organ transplants. The rate of transmission from transfusions and organ transplant is lower with the advent of sensitive blood tests. Sexual transmission is the most common method of transference in the developed world. After inoculation with hepatitis B it is said to be an active infection. This is when the virus is most likely to be transmitted. Upon active infection, the body begins to mount an antibody response. Hepatitis B can be either cured or take on an active carrier state. The former is the most common but a few patients continue to carry hepatitis B. Chronic carriers are at increased risk of infecting others as well as developing liver cancer and cirrhosis. Hepatitis B is easily transmitted for the following two reasons:
- Each mL of blood contains millions of viral copies
- It can survive for days on inanimate objects such as counter tops, tubing, etc.

Precautions with patients with active Hepatitis B
Proper protocol for treating a patient with Hepatitis B:
- Patients with active Hepatitis B should be dialyzed in an isolation area.
- The area could be a separate room or one that is clearly demarcated with caution tape on the floor.
- A nurse dialyzing a Hepatitis B patient should not also dialyze a non-Hepatitis B patient during the same shift.
- Any time a health care worker enters or leaves the isolation area they must change gloves and gowns.
- Gloves and gowns are not permitted to leave the isolation area.
- Dialyzer reuse is never permitted on patients with Hepatitis B and there should be a dedicated Hepatitis B dialysis machine.

Staff screening
Screening for hepatitis B consists of either the HBsAG or anti-HBs blood tests. The former indicates infectivity and the latter indicates immunity. Healthcare workers that are vaccinated and have mounted a response do not need to be screened. Vaccinated healthcare workers who do not mount an adequate response need both HBsAG and anti-HBs every 6 months. Unvaccinated staff should also be screened every 6 months. However, the caveat is in those staff members who are positive for HBsAg or positive for Anti-HBs. The former only need annual HBsAg screening and the latter require no screening at all (they are immune by having recovered from the infection).

Vaccination and monitoring
Hepatitis B is a three series vaccine that is given at baseline, one month and 6 months. There is no guarantee that all persons will mount an appropriate immune response. In these patients a booster vaccine is recommended. There are no recommendations for monitoring hepatitis B immunity after completing the series in health care workers. However, dialysis patients can lose immunity and thus yearly monitoring of Anti-HBs is recommended. If dialysis patients' immunity wane, a booster shot is necessary.

Diagnosing immunity in patients or staff with Hepatitis B
Serum tests are routinely drawn in all health care workers and dialysis patients prior to initiating dialysis. The following blood tests are needed:
- HbsAG (hepatitis B surface antigen)
- Anti-HBc (antibodies against hepatitis B core antigen)
- Anti-HBs (antibodies against hepatitis B surface antigen)

The HBsAG indicates the patient or staff member has active Hepatitis B. Anti-HBs alone indicates immunity against Hepatitis B via vaccination. Anti-HBc along with Anti-HBs indicates that the patient had hepatitis B, have recovered, and are now immune. Patients who are positive for HBsAG are highly infective and must be dialyzed in isolation. Staff and patients with Anti-HBs are immune to hepatitis B and are permitted to work in the isolation area.

Hepatitis C

Hepatitis C used to be known as non-A, non-B hepatitis prior to its discovery. It is an RNA virus that has no present cure. It is transmitted via the blood and is most commonly found in current or ex-intravenous drug users. Other methods of transmission include tattoos and multiple piercings. It is currently treated with interferon and ribavirin. Hepatitis C can cause fulminant hepatic failure early (rare) or liver failure after 20-40 years. It also increases the risk of liver cancer.

HIV

Human Immunodeficiency Virus (HIV) is an RNA virus transmitted via the blood or sexually. It has no cure and vaccines are not available to date. However, progress in highly active antiretroviral therapy (HAART) has made HIV a chronic disease. Patients are surviving in excess of twenty years because of HAART. HIV acts by attacking the body's immune system. Eventually, the immune system becomes so weakened that it cannot fight off the simplest infections or colds. It is also associated with a host of other morbidities. HIV is not easily transmissible. For example, a simple needle stick from a known HIV source carries a 0.3% transmission rate. Factors that increase the chances of transmission include: large bore needle, depth of invasion, and contact of the needle with blood from the source.

Tuberculosis

Tuberculosis (TB) is a bacterium that commonly affects the lungs. While TB can be found in organs outside the pulmonary arena, it is most infective when it attacks the lungs. Transmission of tuberculosis is via respiratory droplets but very difficult. It requires prolonged, intimate exposure to acquire TB (e.g. on a long plane ride, nursing homes, prisons). Dialysis patients are immunocompromised because of their disease. Furthermore, they spend a lot of time in the dialysis center. Thus, TB can be easily transmitted from one patient to another or to staff. Current treatment for TB includes a four-drug regimen which must be taken for two months. The four drugs are isoniazid, rifampin, ethambutol and pyrazinamide. After two months, only isoniazid and rifampin are needed for an additional four months. Choice of drug therapy is dependent on culture sensitivity and local resistance rates.

Tuberculosis screening is done via yearly skin tests. A tuberculin skin test or PPD is placed subdermally and the induration read after 48 hours. Health care workers and dialysis patients have a positive PPD if the induration is greater than 10 mm. If a PPD is positive, a chest x-ray is ordered. A patient with a negative chest x-ray should receive isoniazid prophylaxis for 9 months. A patient with a positive chest x-ray should be treated for active tuberculosis. Patients with active tuberculosis can be dialyzed in respiratory isolation under negative pressure. All staff is required to wear masks prior to entering the isolation room.

Multidrug resistant *Klebsiella* and *Acinetobacter*

Multidrug resistant *Klebsiella* and *Acinetobacter* are also highly resistant gram-negative bacteria. The former is becoming increasingly common in patients with repeated infections following multiple courses of antibiotics. *Acinetobacter* is always an issue for it is difficult to treat regardless of how resistant it may be. Again, patients with these infections require standard precautions and infecting other patients is worrisome.

MRSA and VRE

MRSA and VRE are resistant bacteria to methicillin and vancomycin respectively. Their incidence is increasing and proper barrier protection is warranted to prevent further transmission. Their impact on dialysis patients and staff includes the risk of transmitting resistant bacteria to other patients. Furthermore, they are difficult to treat and thus an outbreak could be disastrous. Patients with MRSA and VRE do not need isolation and standard precautions suffice.

Preparing skin for cannulation of graft or fistula

Described below is the proper preparation of the skin prior to cannulation of the graft or fistula:
- The skin should be palpated for the thrill of the graft or fistula. This is where the needle will be inserted.
- Next, the site is to be washed with either a combination alcohol/chorhexidine gluconate solution or alcohol/povidone solution.
- If either the patient or staff accidentally touches the insertion site after the alcohol preparation, the site is considered contaminated and must be rewashed.
- Clean gloves must be worn by staff throughout the entire process. If the gloves become contaminated at any time, they must be changed prior to cannulation.
- Finally, after cannulation new gloves must be worn between patients.

Infection control techniques used on all catheters

According to the National Kidney Foundation, the following guidelines should be used to lower infection rates:
- The catheter port site should be inspected for signs of infection prior to use before every dialysis session.
- The catheter dressing should be changed with new gauze after each session aseptic techniques must be used which involves the use of gloves for handling of all catheter related procedures and wearing of surgical masks by staff.

Signs of infections or vascular steal phenomena in patients with fistulae and AV grafts

Signs of infection include erythema, swelling, induration, warmth and broken skin. This is usually indicative of a local cellulitis but systemic bacteremia must also be ruled out. Thus, two sets of blood cultures must be sent and intravenous antibiotics covering staphylococcus and streptococcus species begun (usually vancomycin). Alternate access must also be used while the infection resolves. Signs of vascular steal include the following: cool extremity with discoloration and nail bed changes. One should also compare the extremities for warmth, skin color changes and muscle strength. If the site of access differs from the other extremity, vascular steal should be ruled out.

OSHA guidelines for working with chemical disinfectants

OSHA guidelines for personnel safety when using chemical disinfectants include the following:
- Protective gear (eye shields, gloves, and waterproof gowns) should be worn.
- Sufficient ventilation is necessary.
- Splashes on skin or in eyes must be flushed immediately with copious amount of water and medical attention sought.
- A shower and eyewash station must be available.
- All personnel must be well-informed about these hazardous chemicals and their toxicity.
- Printed OSHA requirements and regulations must be available in every dialysis facility.
- Safety Data Sheets (SDS) must be accessible to staff at all times.
- Facility must maintain education records and health monitoring records for all employees.

Dialyzer reprocessing

Reprocessing a dialyzer affects its ability to remove large solutes. Disinfectants that are usually used for dialyzer reprocessing include the following:
- Formaldehyde: second most commonly used disinfectant
- Glutaraldehyde: used in some facilities
- Heat: used in some facilities
- Bleach: decreases membrane clearance of large solutes
- Renalin: used in approximately 70% of facilities to decrease membrane clearance of large solutes such as β2-microglobulin (most commonly used disinfectant)

The labeling requirements are as follows:
- Patient's name: must be used for only one patient
- Number of prior uses
- Date of last reprocessing
- Social security number or birth date
- Additional warning label to notify staff of reuse status of dialyzer-not required, but recommended

Renalin

Either Renalin or formaldehyde is the product of choice most often used for the decontamination process for dialyzers. Renalin is a combination of peracetic acid, acetic acid, and hydrogen peroxide. A 0.5% solution of Renalin is required for disinfecting dialyzers, and it must remain in use for 11 hours. Aqueous formaldehyde (formalin) in a 4% solution must be used for 24 hours at room temperature in order to kill all microorganisms, including viruses and spores. A 1.5% formalin solution must be used at 100° F for a 24 hour period.

Formaldehyde

Potential hazards
Formaldehyde (formalin) is a powerful chemical disinfectant. Formaldehyde (formalin) has been linked to nasal and lung cancer. Airborne concentrates as low as 0.1 parts per million may elicit an irritation response in the nose, eyes, and throat, as well as allergic reactions such as wheezing, cough, and asthma-related symptoms. Whenever this product is used, the air quality must be monitored. The OSHA standard for short-term exposure limit (STEL) is 2 ppm during a 15-minute period. Respiratory training is mandatory for personnel who work with reuse of dialyzers, and they must be fitted for respirators. Annual safety training is required for staff members who use these chemicals.

Formaldehyde exposure
It is critical that the symptoms of formaldehyde reaction are recognized early. If formaldehyde has not been completely removed from the dialyzer, the patient may experience the following:
- Anxiety
- Bitter, peppery taste in mouth
- Burning at the venous needle site
- Numbness around the lips and mouth

- Chest pain
- Back pain
- Shortness of breath

Treatment for formaldehyde reactions are as follows:
- Immediately stop dialysis as hemolysis of red blood cells may occur.
- Remove approximately 10 mL of blood from each needle to ensure the cessation of formaldehyde infusion.

Topical antiseptics

Topical antiseptics are used to clean the skin prior to inserting the cannulation needles. The topical antiseptic solutions most commonly used prior to the insertion of cannulation needles are povidone-iodine and isopropyl alcohol. To cleanse the skin over the proposed injection site, apply the antiseptic with a sterile gauze pad in a circular motion beginning at the proposed site, circling outward until the area cleaned is about 2 inches in diameter. If using the povidone-iodine, allow it to dry before inserting the needle. If isopropyl alcohol is used, insert the needle before the alcohol dries. Follow each manufacturer's instructions for each type of disinfectant to assure effective disinfection.

Governing bodies that establish standards of care for dialysis centers

The Joint Commission on accreditation of Healthcare Organizations (JCAHO) is an independent commission that establishes guidelines for standards of care for all dialysis facilities. Being subject to JCAHO inspections and receiving accreditation is essential for dialysis centers to remain open and for reimbursement from Centers for Medicare and Medicaid Services (CMS). Finally, CMS and state laws also play a role in establishing health care guidelines as well as water supply maintenance and cleanliness.

Patient Rights and Regulatory Guidelines

Dialysis facility structure

A typical dialysis facility is headed by a Director. This person is usually a nephrologist, albeit a multidisciplinary approach is taken. The nephrologist is chiefly involved with managing dialysis patients' renal disease and is responsible for writing dialysis orders. The dialysis nurse is the person responsible for the direct care of patients. They operate and manage the dialysis treatment, administer medications and collect blood samples for pre and post-dialysis values. Frequently, there is a nurse manager or nurse practitioner who oversees the nursing staff. Their main function is to work with nephrologists, nurses and other members of the team to help coordinate and facilitate care. Some dialysis centers also employ a dialysis technician. They are involved with dialysis equipment setup and maintenance. Finally, renal dietitians and social workers round up the major players in dialysis care. Dietitians help patients and their families organize renal responsive diets with particular attention to ensuring this population is not malnourished. Social workers aid patients and their families deal with psychological and other ethical issues.

HIPAA

HIPAA stands for health insurance portability and accountability act. This act was passed in 1996. It ensures patient privacy. All medical records and access to those records are available to health care professionals only. Moreover, the health care professional must access those records only in the interest of caring for the patient. If the health care worker is not actively caring for the patient, it is a HIPAA violation to access that patient's medical record. Furthermore, the sharing of medical information between health care personnel in a manner not specifically aimed at patient care (e.g. water cooler discussion) is prohibited. The information protected includes all information contained in paper charts, electronic medical records, laboratory results or oral communication.

Rights of patient prior to and after beginning hemodialysis

Foremost, patients have the right to decline dialysis provided a clinician has illustrated to them the risks, benefits and alternatives to refusing treatment. Patients must also consent prior to beginning any dialysis treatment, including transferring from one facility to another. Other patient rights include:
- To be informed about their disease and prognosis
- To be informed about the risks of treatment as well as the risks of withholding treatment
- To be informed about alternatives to treatment,
- To have the final say regarding their choice of treatment

Advance directive

An advanced directive is a written document outlining the type of treatment a patient would want to receive should they lose the capacity to make decisions. An advanced directive can be as detailed as denying CPR or intubation or as general as assigning a health care proxy. A health care proxy can be anyone the patient assigns. The proxy is allowed to make treatment decisions for the patient as long as the patient does not have capacity. The proxy cannot make decisions which are contrary to the patient's wishes or written directive.

Process, standard, and clinical indicator

The terms outlined are defined below:
- Process—A flow of procedures in carrying out an activity. For example, in order to prepare a patient for dialysis one needs the orders, proper dialysate, predialysis checking of the machine, dialyzer, etc. This is a process to get the patient ready for dialysis.
- Standards—Minimum parameters set by governing bodies to which all personnel are held accountable. For example, the American Nephrology Nurses Association sets standards for specific patient outcomes such as how to properly cannulate a graft or fistula.
- Clinical indicator—Measures used to evaluate patient outcomes. These are metrics outlined by governing bodies such as JCAHO. An example would be how many venous punctures are used to cannulate a graft or fistula.

KDOQI

The National Kidney Foundation has launched the Kidney Disease Outcomes Quality Initiative (KDOQI). It provides evidence-based guidelines for all dialysis personnel for all stages of chronic kidney disease. This initiative was first launched in 1997 and has ongoing research projects and recommendations for all to use. Currently, the National Kidney Foundation has 11 KDOQI guidelines and it is accepted practice to adhere to these guidelines.

CQI and TQM

CQI stands for continuous quality improvement. It operates under the umbrella of total quality management (TQM). CQI is an ongoing active process in which dialysis centers ask the following: how can we improve patient care? CQI implicates all types of quality outcomes from disease specific to dialysis procedure specific. The key to CQI is to keep it patient focused. CQI operates under TQM. TQM is upper management's commitment towards improving dialysis care and quality. Initiatives to improve care include vaccinations, infection rates, water quality control, etc.

Benchmark and outcome

A benchmark provides a reference point for dialysis facilities. A benchmark could be national or local. For example, how does dialysis facility A compare with dialysis facility B in total mortality or infection rates? Benchmarks are useful in comparing how one is doing relative to others. An outcome is a clinically relevant metric used after some action has taken place. For example, a dialysis facility may decide to lower the number of infection rates by 50% by implementing new infection control guidelines. After implementing the guidelines the infection rate is measured and compared to prior values.

Professional boundaries

Professional boundaries must be maintained between healthcare workers and dialysis patients. "Professional boundaries" refer to the self-imposed restraints that the dialysis staff must maintain in order to achieve a therapeutic relationship with their patients. The National Council of State Boards of Nursing, Inc. defines this as "the spaces between the nurse's power and the client's vulnerability". Since dialysis patients may be under the care of the dialysis staff several times a week over a period of several years, a close relationship may develop. The healthcare worker should not overstep these boundaries by spending time with the patient after normal working hours, entering any business arrangements, socializing, having any sexual relationship, or accepting gifts or any type from the patient or family members. Intimate relationship with a patient is considered misconduct and a serious violation of the Nurse Practice Acts in most states.

Peritoneal Dialysis

Advantages and disadvantages of HD and PD for the ESRD patient with diabetes

The diabetic patient who undergoes in-center HD treatment has these advantages:
- Frequent medical observation
- Less loss of protein during dialysis treatment

The disadvantages are as follows:
- Higher risk of vascular access complications
- Risk of predialysis hyperkalemia
- Increase chance of hypotension during treatment

The advantages for the diabetic patient who chooses PD are as follows:
- Better glycemic control, especially with intraperitoneal insulin
- Better cardiovascular tolerance
- Better potassium control
- Vascular access is not required

The disadvantages are as follows:
- Peritonitis
- Protein loss
- Increase in intraabdominal pressure complications, for example gastroparesis

Peritoneal dialysis

Peritoneal dialysis uses the peritoneal cavity, which is approximately equal to the body's surface area, as a reservoir in which the dialysate is infused via a catheter. The peritoneum acts as a semipermeable membrane through which surplus body fluid and solutes, including uremic toxins, are removed (ultrafiltrate).

Peritoneal dialysis is the process by which dialysis can occur using the peritoneal membrane. Hypertonic dialysate filled with dextrose is infused into the peritoneum via an indwelling catheter. The dialysate fills the abdominal cavity. The peritoneum serves as the semipermeable membrane allowing for urea, potassium and other toxins to diffuse into the dialysate. Moreover, the dialysate is hypertonic which permits excess body water to diffuse into the peritoneum (ultrafiltration). The fluid is than drained and this entire process is known as an exchange.

Peritoneal dialysis allows the patient a simpler, home-based therapy with little need for special water systems. The equipment is easy to set up and use. The two types of PD are continuous ambulatory peritoneal dialysis (CAPD) where the patient performs manual exchanges 4-5 times a day and continuous cycling peritoneal dialysis (CCPD) where the exchanges are done while the patient is sleeping.

Patients who often favor PD include the following:
- Children and infants
- Patients with severe cardiovascular disease
- Patients with diabetes
- Patients who prefer the freedom
- Patients who prefer home dialysis, but have no one to assist them

Disadvantages
While peritoneal dialysis offers patients the advantage of at home dialysis, it does come with some disadvantages. The first is an increase in malnutrition. The peritoneal membrane with frequent exchanges allows for excess protein loss. Protein malnutrition is very common in these patients. Moreover, the dextrose in the dialysate is reabsorbed. The dextrose causes hypertriglyceridemia and worsens obesity and diabetes. Finally, adequacy of dialysis is not as good when compared to hemodialysis. In order to comply with the K/DOQI guidelines for adequacy, patients are often asked to perform more exchanges with larger volumes each day.

Advantages for elderly patients
The advantages of PD for the elderly patient consist of the following:
- No time, effort, or expense invested in traveling to the dialysis center
- Maintenance of control of their therapy, which promotes independence
- Preservation of usual lifestyle
- Ability to set own schedule
- Lack of need for vascular access, which is important because many elderly patients have poor peripheral vessels
- Maintenance of therapies, blood chemistry levels, and fluid status
- Slow, continuous therapy possible, preferable for correction of brain electrophysiologic and cognitive function abnormalities
- Less rigid dietary and fluid restrictions

Disadvantages for elderly patients
Some of the disadvantages of using PD as the mode of choice for the elderly patient include the following:
- The incidence of complications, such as dementia, hernias, peritonitis, *Staphylococcus epidermis,* and abdominal and catheter leaks all are higher in the elderly population on PD.
- If patient needs significant ultrafiltration, the dialysate glucose concentration may depress the appetite and lead to malnutrition even if dry weight is stable; dextrose provides calories but little nutrition (this may be hard to diagnose initially).
- There is a loss of social experience. Interaction with others takes place in the dialysis center.

Advantages and disadvantages of treating diabetics
The dialysate contains glucose, which is used as an osmotic gradient for diffusion of urea and other solutes. The glucose is also absorbed by the peritoneum and can elevate serum sugar. Thus, dialysate is frequently given with insulin in diabetics. The advantage of insulin with the dialysate is having a basal steady state of insulin to keep glucose fluctuations at a minimum. The disadvantage of insulin is the risk of hypoglycemia. Furthermore, dialyzing diabetics via the peritoneum puts them at risk of absorbing too much dextrose and elevating serum glucose for prolonged periods.

Peritoneal membrane

The peritoneal membrane is the term used to describe the lining of the abdominal cavity and pelvic walls including the diaphragm (parietal peritoneum) and the covering of the abdominal organs (visceral peritoneum). In males, it is completely sealed; in females, it opens into the Fallopian tubes and ovaries.

Exchange process

The peritoneal membrane maintains contact with an abundance of blood vessels that supply the abdominal organs. In peritoneal dialysis, the dialysate is infused by means of a catheter, permitted to remain in the peritoneal cavity for a set amount of time, and then removed (effluent). This procedure is termed "an exchange." An osmotic gradient is created by using dextrose in the dialysate, which causes the shift of water into the peritoneal cavity. The surplus of water is removed when the effluent is drained. The process of diffusion causes electrolytes and uremic toxins to be removed from areas of higher concentration (bloodstream) to the area of lower concentration (peritoneal cavity). Low-molecular-weight solutes are "dragged" when solute removal is enhanced by use of a hypertonic dialysate, which increases ultrafiltration (UF) by means of convective transport.

Contraindications to peritoneal dialysis

There are many reasons to not initiate peritoneal dialysis in patients. Foremost, they need the support structure at home. Second, they must be open and willing to learn a new method of caring for themselves including troubleshooting (signs of infection, etc.). They must also have the manual dexterity and vision to carry out the requirements of peritoneal dialysis. Finally, clinical contraindications include peritoneal adhesions or fibrosis, abdominal neoplasm, documented poor peritoneal equilibration test, current or recurrent peritonitis and communication between the peritoneal and thoracic cavities.

Continuous ambulatory peritoneal dialysis

Continuous ambulatory peritoneal dialysis (CAPD) is a dialysis method where the patient performs approximately 4-6 exchanges throughout the day. The term ambulatory differentiates this type of dialysis from automated peritoneal dialysis (continuous dialysis at night). The exchanges are carried out as per the nephrologist's orders. The dialysate enters the peritoneal cavity and sits there to allow for diffusion. After a predetermined time, the fluid is drained. The main drawback to CAPD is that one must perform an exchange every 4-6 hours.

Automated peritoneal dialysis

Automated peritoneal dialysis occurs when a machine automatically performs the exchanges. The machine is preprogrammed to deliver a set amount of fluid with timed frequencies. The dialysate used is prescribed by the nephrologist. The machine also warms the dialysate prior to infusion. The advantage to automated peritoneal dialysis is that it can be done at night without interfering with the patient's daily activities. Finally, a daytime dwelling dialysate can be left over to help clear larger molecules. The patient does not perform an exchange during the day but rather carries the excess dialysate fluid with them.

There are four types of automated peritoneal dialysis:
- Continuous cycling peritoneal dialysis—Three to five nightly exchanges with a daytime infusion to aid in molecular clearance.
- Nocturnal intermittent peritoneal dialysis—Three to five nightly exchanges with no daytime infusion. This is prescribed in patients who hyperabsorb the dextrose solution, suffer from congestive heart failure or have hernias and chronic low back pain.
- Intermittent peritoneal dialysis—Exchanges are performed three to five times per week. There is no left over dialysate in the peritoneum between exchanges. This is a more cost effective method to dialysis and is also used in patients with residual renal function.
- Tidal peritoneal dialysis—Dialysate is initially infused into the peritoneum. After a predetermined time in the peritoneal cavity most of the dialysate is drained leaving some fluid behind. The fluid acts to increase clearance. When the next exchange occurs, a new dialysate is introduced (tidal dialysis). The cycle than repeats.

Peritoneal dialysate solutions

The dialysate used contains dextrose (glucose) to facilitate the osmotic gradient necessary for dialysis. The dialysate also contains sodium, chloride, calcium, magnesium and lactate to approximate the extracellular electrolyte concentrations. Only potassium is absent or in lower concentrations to facilitate total body K removal. The solutions come in different dextrose concentrations: 1.5%, 2.5% and 4.25%. The increasing dextrose concentrations help facilitate a greater exchange. Finally, icodextrin is a new dialysate solution that does not contain dextrose. Instead, icodextrin employs a glucose polymer and aids in greater fluid removal.

Commercially available solutions

These solutions are created to be similar to extracellular fluid with the exception of potassium. Some of the commercially available peritoneal dialysis solutions are as follows:
- Dianeal PD-2
- Dianeal PD-1
- Dianeal Low Ca
- Icodextrin (Extraneal) does not contain dextrose, uses a starch derived osmotic agent
- Delflex

Potassium is not used in these dialysate solutions because many patients are hyperkalemic. Potassium may be added to the solution (2-4 mEq/L) if needed or an oral supplement may be prescribed. The more hypertonic the dialysate solution is, the greater the ultrafiltration that occurs. Dextrose is the ingredient that provides the osmotic gradient between plasma and dialysate facilitating the fluid and solute removal.

Icodextrin

Icodextrin (Extraneal) is a dialysis solution that does not contain dextrose. Instead, it uses a starch based osmotic agent made from glucose polymers. This starch based solution allows for enhanced fluid removal from the blood during peritoneal dialysis, increases small solute clearance, and lowers the incidence of net negative ultrafiltration. Icodextrin is prescribed for use once in a 24-hour period via a long dwelling exchange lasting 8-16 hours. This product is contraindicated for those individuals with cornstarch allergies and those with glycogen storage diseases. Skin rash is the most commonly seen adverse effect with sterile peritonitis, hypertension, influenza-like symptoms, headache, and abdominal pain experienced by some patients.

Peritoneal dialysis catheter

A surgeon usually inserts a peritoneal dialysis catheter during a laparoscopy or laparotomy procedure. The usual exit site of is in midquadrant avoiding scars, skinfolds, or beltline. Catheters are either straight or coiled and have one or two cuffs. The coiled catheters are frequently preferred due to their minimal migration from the original insertion location and their lack of outflow problems. Coiled catheters also seem to cause less discomfort for the patient due to the configuration that keeps the tip of the catheter away from the peritoneal membrane. The cuffs, which are made of Dacron polyester or velour, allow ingrowth of tissue which stabilizes the catheter. In double cuffed catheters, the internal cuff is located in the rectus muscle with the external cuff placed in the subcutaneous tissue.

The four types of PD catheters used for long-term placement in the peritoneum include the following:
- Straight Tenckhoff catheter
- Curled Tenckhoff catheter
- Toronto western catheter
- Swan-neck (Missouri) catheter

Catheter "break-in" refers to the amount of time from when the chronic catheter is placed in the peritoneum until tissue ingrowth and healing have occurred. The goals during this "break-in" period of about six weeks are to promote healing and prevent complications such as dialysate leaks, infections or catheter obstruction. Full-volume dialysis should be avoided for a minimum of 10-14 days to allow healing to occur.

Factors that influence ultrafiltration and solute clearance

The following factors are implicated in clearance and ultrafiltration:
- Permeability of the peritoneal membrane (more permeable = better clearance)
- Volume of the exchange (higher volume = greater clearance)
- Dialysate glucose concentration (higher concentration = better clearance and fluid removal)
- Dwell time (longer times allow for more diffusion)
- Molecular size (small molecules are cleared more efficiently)

Other forms of at home dialysis

The other main form of at home dialysis is home hemodialysis. This is rarely used today but was popular in the early 1970s. It is hemodialysis carried out by the patient at home. Problems with home hemodialysis include gaining access, sterile environment and having adequate support. The dialysis at home is usually a slow dialysis or a form of CRRT. This helps decrease the incidence of hypotension and ensures a more adequate dialysis.

Peritoneal Dialysis Complications

The most common complications include:
- Peritonitis
- Exit site infection
- Fibrin formation
- Tunnel infection
- Hemoperitoneum (blood in peritoneum)
- Inflow/outflow obstruction
- Pneumoperitoneum (air in peritoneum)
- Dialysate leak
- Hernia
- Pain on inflow

Exit site infections

Exit site infections occur when the skin flora (staph and strep) infect the exit site of the catheter. Signs of exit site infections include purulent drainage, skin induration and erythema along with abdominal pain. Exit site infections increase the risk of bacteria migrating into the peritoneum causing peritonitis. Treatment includes intraperitoneal along with systemic oral or intravenous antibiotics. Local care should also be increased with dressing changes occurring more frequently. Catheter removal may be necessary.

Peritonitis

Peritonitis is the most common complication of peritoneal dialysis. The indwelling catheter along with any exchanges increases the risk of introducing bacteria. Patients with peritonitis will present with abdominal pain, fever and nausea/vomiting. Laboratory studies will reveal elevated peritoneal white blood cell counts. Treatment includes intraperitoneal antibiotics to cover both gram-positive and gram-negative organisms.

Y-system

The Y-system is a set of connecting tubes and double bags, one of dialysate and the other empty. A stem connects to the peripheral dialysis catheter and transfer set with the afferent limb connected to the PD dialysate solution bag and the efferent limb attached to the empty drainage bag. There are clamps on both lines (limbs) to control the rate and direction of fluid flow allowing drainage or infusion. Priming the main stem with PD solution and allowing this solution to drain into the drainage bag instead of into the peritoneum has dramatically decreased the incidence of peritonitis.

Tunnel infections

Pathophysiology and treatment of tunnel infections is explained below:
- Tunnel infections must be differentiated from exit site infections.
- Tunnel infections are subcutaneous and not readily visible.
- Tunnel infections are also not intraperitoneal and should not be confused with peritonitis.

- Signs of tunnel infections include erythema with underlying inflammation and swelling of the cuff.
- Treatment includes intravenous and intraperitoneal antibiotics.
- Tunnel infections also increase the risk of peritonitis.

Fibrin formation

Fibrin formation occurs following peritonitis or a local inflammation from a previous infection. Fibrin clots or strands form during inflammatory processes and occur because of decreased clot degradation during the process. It is diagnosed when fibrin strands (white strands) are seen in the effluent. Treatment includes heparin being added to the dialysate.

Inflow/outflow obstructions

Inflow/outflow obstructions occur when fibrin clots form or catheter positioning changes. It is diagnosed when dialysate will neither enter nor exit the catheter. Treatment is usually with heparin flushes to break up the clots. If that does not work than plain films are taken and the catheter repositioned. Finally, the catheter may need to be replaced.

Hemoperitoneum

Hemoperitoneum means blood in the peritoneal cavity. The most common causes include retrograde menstruation, trauma with introducing the dialysis catheter, ruptured ovarian cysts and peritonitis. It is diagnosed when blood tinged or bright red blood is seen in the effluent. Hemoperitoneum is usually self-limiting but treatment includes frequent flushes with saline to prevent clot formation.

Dialysate leak

A dialysate leak occurs when there is room around the catheter site or in the subcutaneous tissue for the dialysate to enter. Patients with a dialysate leak will often have increased abdominal pressure with clear fluid draining around the exit site or edema. It is diagnosed with a dextrostick and treated with cessation of peritoneal dialysis until the exit site heals or is resutured. Dialysate volume can also be decreased with each exchange to facilitate less fluid loss.

Pneumoperitoneum

Pneumoperitoneum means air in the peritoneal cavity. Each exchange will introduce some air into the peritoneal cavity. However, excess air can cause bowel obstruction and peritonitis. Pneumoperitoneum is diagnosed with excess bloating and shoulder pain. Plain abdominal films will confirm the diagnosis. Treatment involves draining the patient in Trendelenburg or knee-chest position. Moreover, looking for air leaks in the catheter is also important to rule loose connections.

Pain on inflow

When dialysate is infused into the peritoneal cavity it can be painful. This is secondary to catheter migration near the peritoneal wall, acidic dialysate or rapid infusion. Treatment includes slower infusion rates, application of local anesthetics, and addition of bicarbonate or catheter change.

Hernias

Hernias occur when the dialysate fluid is introduced into the peritoneal cavity. The fluid-filled cavity will expand and any weakness in the abdominal wall musculature will be exploited by bowel. Ventral hernias are common. Most often surgery is not required for treatment as long as the hernia is readily reducible. However, surgery is the only definitive treatment.

Inflow and outflow problems

Peritoneal dialysis patients may experience inflow or outflow problems and may inadvertently get air in the abdomen. The catheter may become obstructed due to fibrin, blood, or omentum occluding the opening. Inflow and outflow problems may also be caused by the catheter's position, due to its migration out of the pelvis. Loculation caused by adhesions or constipation may also be considered as possible causes of obstruction of flow. Treatment options include the following:
- Relieving constipation
- X-ray for internal catheter kink
- Inspect catheter for external kinks
- Irrigate catheter with heparinized saline or a thrombolytic
- Reposition or replace catheter
- Peritoneogram with contrast medium to identify loculation

Air may enter the abdomen via loose connections or air in the system. The patient may complain of shoulder pain and peritoneal eosinophilia may be seen. Intervention includes draining the patient of the effluent and placing the patient in the knee-chest or Trendelenburg position. The air will be absorbed over time. Tighten all connections and inspect lines for presence of air.

Negatives associated with PD

Some of the negatives associated with peritoneal dialysis (PD) include protein malnutrition and inadequate dialysis. The protein malnutrition results from the loss of amino acids and protein in the dialysate. The appetite is decreased due to the glucose load absorbed from the dialysis. This frequently results in hypertriglyceridemia, which causes weight gain from the caloric increase. Once residual renal function ceases, many patients are inadequately dialyzed using peritoneal dialysis. This results in the ESRD patient changing modes of dialysis from PD to HD in order to achieve optimal dialysis results.

Peritoneal dialysis in children

In children, peritoneal dialysis is the most commonly used method of chronic dialysis therapy. Most children use a cycling machine for overnight ADP. Complications of PD in children include the following:
- Catheter obstruction by omentum - usually prevented surgically by removing or trimming the omentum
- Inguinal and umbilical hernias - surgeon should review treatment
- Leakage around the catheter or exit site - usually indicates that the catheter has been used before the PD tract had sufficiently healed
- Peritonitis - prevention using excellent aseptic technique, comprehensive training for all caregivers, and closed-line delivery systems

- Growth problems due to reduced appetite with increased catabolic demands - monitoring and improving nutrition, correcting acidosis, and assessing bone disease and growth, using human growth hormone if indicated
- Hypertension is seen less frequently in children than in adults, but when severe, may require a prophylactic nephrectomy.

Interventions

Accessing the peritoneum for peritoneal dialysis

Peritoneal dialysis is done via a catheter, which is inserted near the umbilicus. This is a bedside procedure and there are various catheters. Catheters are inserted into the peritoneal cavity with tunneled cuffs to provide an adequate seal in the subcutaneous tissue. The tunneled cuffs also provide a barrier for invading infections. Catheters must remain in place for 10-14 days before being used. This allows for granulation and healing.

Peritoneal equilibration test

The peritoneal equilibration test is used to determine peritoneal membrane permeability. First, the patient's peritoneum is infused with 2.5% dialysate. Then dialysate samples of urea, glucose and creatinine are taken at 0, 2, 4 and 12 hours. The serum is also sampled for urea and glucose at 2 hours. The ratio of dialysate to peritoneal creatinine concentration is plotted against a standard chart. The same applies for glucose concentrations at 2 and 4 hours over glucose at 0 hours. The ratios are plotted against established standards and the peritoneal dialysate is adjusted accordingly.

Determining peritoneal dialysis adequacy

The peritoneal equilibration test allows nephrologists to adjust peritoneal dialysate regimens and give insight to permeability. It does not, however, yield adequacy. Adequacy in dialysis is determined by the formula Kt/V. Kt/V is obtained by a 24-hour urine collection along with effluent (dialysis clearance). The current targets for adequacy as defined by the National Kidney Foundation are: continuous ambulatory peritoneal dialysis - $Kt/V > 2.0$, continuous cycling peritoneal dialysis - $Kt/V > 2.1$ and nocturnal intermittent peritoneal dialysis - $Kt/V > 2.2$.

Medications administered with peritoneal dialysis

Dialysate is the fluid administered into the abdominal cavity to perform peritoneal dialysis. This is available in 1.5%, 2.5%, and 4.25 percent dextrose concentration. The higher the concentration of dextrose, the more fluid and waste will move into the abdominal cavity. Some of the regular medications that are taken on a daily basis by patients with peritoneal dialysis may include ACE inhibitors and diuretics. ACE inhibitors are used to treat hypertension and help to protect kidney function. Diuretics help the body to eliminate excess fluid and sodium. Peritoneal dialysis patients may also be taking vitamin D and phosphorous for bone strength. Vitamin D is produced by the kidneys, so patients on dialysis may not be producing the amount required to maintain bone strength. Iron may also be necessary if the patient is anemic. A hormone that is produced in the kidneys that stimulates red blood cell production, erythropoietin, may also need to be given for anemia. With kidney failure, it is very important that patients are educated on not taking any medications that have not been prescribed by their physician.

Alternatives to administering erythropoietin in patients on peritoneal dialysis

In patients on peritoneal dialysis, another method of administering erythropoietin is via the peritoneum. This is reserved for patients who do not tolerate the intravenous or subcutaneous route of administration. The peritoneum must be dry or with minimal dialysate. Moreover, the injection dose is usually increased by about 50% in those patients so as to achieve adequate levels of erythropoietin. The major drawback with giving intraperitoneal erythropoietin is lower absorption and the possibility of peritonitis. Anytime the peritoneal cavity is invaded, the prospect of bacterial or other form of peritonitis is increased substantially.

Limitations of intraperitoneal erythropoietin injections

Intraperitoneal injections of erythropoietin require higher dosing than subcutaneous injections. The requirement is usually about 50 percent more and is necessary to ensure an adequate level of erythropoietin enters the system. Peritoneal injections of erythropoietin are also limited by decreased absorption by the peritoneal membrane and by the amount of fluid in the peritoneal cavity. Fluid in the peritoneal cavity acts to dilute the erythropoietin and will decrease its absorption. Therefore, it is always recommended that patients getting intraperitoneal erythropoietin should have a "dry" peritoneum or less than 50 ml of dialysate. Excess dialysate fluid will hinder proper absorption and decrease erythropoietin's efficacy.

Patient education before peritoneal dialysis

Once a decision has been made that peritoneal dialysis is right for the patient, a catheter is placed through the abdominal wall. The patient will need to be educated on caring for the catheter and cleaning around the catheter site to decrease the risk of infection. There is a risk of developing a hernia at the catheter site if there is straining to move the bowels, so they need to receive education on constipation prevention. Once the catheter site has healed, after about 2 weeks, education begins on how to perform peritoneal dialysis at home. The solution used, the dwell time (how long the fluid remains in the abdomen), and how to drain the fluid will need to be taught based on the type of dialysate used. The patient also needs to be educated on when to contact their healthcare provider with any problems. The development of abdominal pain, redness or swelling at the catheter site, cloudy dialysate fluid, or fever may indicate peritonitis, which needs to be treated urgently.

Home peritoneal dialysis
Outpatient training a patient for home peritoneal dialysis should be done once the patient has recovered from the catheter insertion surgery, which usually takes at least 2 weeks. An additional person who would be available to assist the patient at home, if needed, should also attend these sessions. The content must be customized to the patient's education level and learning abilities and should include the following:
- Basics of normal kidney function
- Effects of renal failure
- Mechanics of peritoneal dialysis
- Importance of aseptic technique
- Maintenance and care of catheter and exit site
- Record-keeping: body weight, blood pressure, treatments performed
- CAPD exchange procedures

- Use of a cycler if on APD
- Choice of dialysate solutions
- Recognition of signs and symptoms of infections
- Peritonitis and treatments
- Medications
- Ordering of supplies
- Dietary counseling
- Management of complications

Psychosocial considerations when considering peritoneal dialysis at home

Some of the psychosocial issues to be considered when making the decision to use peritoneal dialysis at home are as follows:
- Patient's ability and motivation for self-care
- Employment or school requirements, scheduling conflicts
- Educational background
- Health beliefs
- Family and community support system
- Patient's state of mind, comprehension
- History of compliance with medical treatment
- Travel distance from dialysis facility
- Physical characteristics of home, availability of water source, electricity, phone, storage room for supplies, cleanliness
- Availability of additional caregiver, such as spouse, relative, friend

PD quality assurance indicators

The goal of quality assurance should be continuous improvement. The Joint Commission on the Accreditation of Healthcare Organizations (JCAHO) and the Centers for Medicare and Medicaid (CMS) issue mandates that are implemented on a regional level by the ESRD networks to improve the care of the PD patient. Some quality assurance indicators are as follows:
- Incidence of treatment-related infections, such as peritonitis and exit site/tunnel infections
- Incidence of catheter complications, pericatheter leaks, migration, obstruction requiring replacement, and holes or cracks in catheters
- Patient morbidity, number of hospitalization days per year and cause of hospitalizations, and mortality
- Attainment of adequacy goals
- Constant review and revision of policies and procedures to improve quality of patient care

Transplant

Patients not considered candidates for renal transplantation surgery

Patients who cannot currently be considered for renal transplantation include the following:
- Those with active infections
- Patients with ongoing malignancies
- Patients who are current substance abusers
- Patients who are unable to adhere to medication schedules

Patients who may be considered, but whose transplantations are relatively contraindicated, include the following:
- Patients who are very young or over 65
- Patients with severe disease processes
- Patients with no family or other support mechanisms
- Patients with severe mental or psychological issues

HIV patients were not considered as candidates for renal transplantation surgery in the past because of the effect of the immunosuppressant drugs on the HIV infection. There currently is no policy that states patients who are HIV+ cannot receive transplants. Studies are being conducted at the University of Pittsburgh transplant center to determine the safety of liver and kidney transplants in the HIV+ patient.

Kidney donation

The two sources for kidneys used in transplantation are living donors and deceased donors. There are only two requirements for a living donor to be considered as the source of a kidney. The donor must give voluntary informed consent and must be completely healthy. In order for a deceased person to be used as a kidney donor, the following requirements must be met:
- The patient must have had irreversible brain damage.
- Consent must have been given by the next of kin.
- The body must have been kept functioning by artificial ventilation and medications.
- The kidney must be recovered by organ recovery team.
- The kidney must go to a regional tissue and organ bank as per national guidelines to be distributed to a proper recipient.
- No expense is incurred by the donor family.

Immunological basis of organ transplantation

The immune system guards the body against attacks from foreign invaders by identifying and destroying them. Anything that produces the 'identify and destroy' response by the immune system is termed an "antigen." Transplant researchers have identified two main antigen systems: blood groups (ABO), and human leukocyte antigen (HLA). The blood groups (ABO) are the first consideration when determining organ compatibility with the recipient with potential recipients divided by blood type. Rh (rhesus) factor does not affect solid organ transplantation. The HLA system comes from genes found in six locations on chromosomes. When tissue is introduced with unrecognized HLA genes, the rejection process begins. The most important components of the immune system are T-cells, which distinguish the tissue as foreign and start the rejection process, and B-cell lymphocytes, which recognize the foreign antigen and produce antibodies to destroy it.

Advantages and disadvantages to kidney transplants

The major advantage to a kidney transplant is the increase in quality of life. Patients no longer have to attend thrice weekly hemodialysis or perform daily peritoneal exchanges at home. The lack of dependence on dialysis allows patients more independence and a greater sense of well-being. Transplant recipients also have a longer survival rate in contrast to dialysis patients. The disadvantage to transplantation is the lifelong dependence on immunosuppressive agents. Immunosuppression leaves patients susceptible to opportunistic infections including candida and possibly cancer. Moreover, the regimen of immunosuppressive agents can be both costly and complicated. Adverse effects from medications are quite common.

Immunologic response to transplanted kidney

The transplanted kidney is a foreign body. The body's immune system recognizes antigens on the surface of the kidney as foreign. The immune system will defend itself by attacking the invading tissue. It specifically recognizes the human leukocyte antigen (HLA) and the ABO blood type as foreign. Thus, prior to transplantation a donor's blood type as well as HLA must match the recipient. Yet, even with matching antigens the immune system will react to the new kidney as a foreign invader. The role of immunosuppressants is to curtail the immune system's response. By suppressing the immunologic reaction, transplant nephrologists hope to preserve the new kidney's structure and function.

Contraindications to receiving kidney transplant

The contraindications include:
- Infection
- Cancer
- Substance abuse (alcohol or drugs)
- Noncompliance
- Severe comorbidities

Panel reactive antibody

Panel reactive antibody (PRA) is the process of taking the recipient's blood and mixing it with random donors' lymph cells. The patient's serum will cross react with some donors while not reacting with others. The percent reaction defines the PRA level. The higher the percentage of reactivity, the less compatible a recipient will be to a donor. Therefore, if a patient has a high PRA level and they are matched with someone, they are given precedence. Patients with lower PRA scores will be more forgiving in accepting a larger range of potential kidneys.

Crossmatching

Crossmatching is the process of mixing recipient's blood with the donor's lymph cells to check for cross reactivity. First, samples from a recipient's blood are taken. Second, lymph cells are taken from the donor. The samples are then mixed. If the recipient's blood reacts to the lymph cells (attacks them), than that patient cannot receive the kidney. Although the recipient may not have been exposed to the donor's cells before, immune systems have a large range of antigen recognition.

The immune system can recognize an antigen it has never seen before and attack it. This phenomenon occurs if that antigen is similar in structure to another antigen that the patient was previously exposed to.

Rejection

There are three general types of rejection:
- Hyperacute—Humoral based rejection. Preformed antibodies immediately attack the transplanted kidney within minutes. This is catastrophic and the transplant must be removed before it becomes infected. This is usually prevented with proper cross matching.
- Acute rejection—Cellular based rejection. T cells recognize the foreign kidney and start mounting an immune response. This rejection takes place within the first few months after transplantation.
- Chronic rejection—Humoral based rejection. This happens in all transplanted organs with time. The body forms antibodies against the transplant and slowly eats away at it. This is defined by a slow decline in kidney function with fibrosis noted in a biopsy.

Cellular and humoral rejection
There are two types of rejection: cellular and humoral.
- Cellular refers to T lymphocytes directly attacking the transplanted kidney. This is known as cell-to-cell combat.
- Humoral refers to antibodies attacking the transplanted kidney. The antibodies are released from B cells and like missiles attack the transplant. Immunosuppressive medicines target the actions of both T and B lymphocytes to limit the number and efficacy of attacks launched.

Diagnosis and treatment
Rejection is commonly picked up by rising creatinine and oliguria. However, care must be taken to rule out other insults to the transplanted kidney including: medication induced, prerenal azotemia, obstruction, etc.
- Hyperacute rejection—Diagnosed immediately. The kidney quickly becomes necrotic with symptoms of a rapidly rising creatinine, fever, oliguria and pain. Treatment is to remove the kidney.
- Acute rejection—Diagnosed with oliguria, fever and tenderness over the transplant sight. This is the most common rejection and immunosuppressive agents are largely targeting this type of rejection. If the addition of steroids along with other immunosuppressive agents does not resolve the issue, the transplant may need to be removed.
- Chronic rejection—Diagnosed with a slowly rising creatinine. It is usually a diagnosis of exclusion and a biopsy is necessary. Only mycophenolate mofetil has been shown to lower chronic rejection rates.

Surgical procedure involved with kidney transplants

The transplanted kidney is placed in the iliac fossa. The iliac fossa is chosen to facilitate ease of placing the transplanted kidney as well as easier access in case it should be removed. Moreover, the iliac fossa is near the internal iliac artery and vein as well as the bladder to aid in the anastomosis of vessels and ureter. The transplanted renal artery and vein are anastomosed with their respective internal iliac artery and vein. The transplanted ureter is attached to the bladder.

The procedure usually lasts from 2-4 hours and the entire hospital course is approximately 3-5 days.

Pre-transplant work up for patients

Patients who are eligible for transplants should be referred to transplant centers. Transplant centers are equipped with multidisciplinary teams consisting of surgeons, transplant nephrologists, social workers, and nurse coordinators. They assist the patient and their family through the process. Preoperative workup includes the following:
- Complete cardiopulmonary assessment to ensure optimal or near optimal heart and lung function
- Signs of infection anywhere in the body
- Age-related cancer screening
- Psychological evaluation to screen for depression/anxiety as well as substance abuse

Dialysis after kidney transplant

A transplanted kidney is often slow to respond to its new environment. It may take days to produce adequate urine. In fact, there is no guarantee that a transplanted kidney will ever respond but the benefits far outweigh that risk. While the transplanted kidney is responding dialysis may be necessary. Dialysis in the post-operative patient must be careful so as not to compromise the new kidney. Thus, no anticoagulation or hypotension during dialysis can be tolerated.

Precautions
The most important part of post transplant dialysis is to ensure the safety of the transplanted organs. Any insult to the fragile transplanted kidney could place the whole process in jeopardy. Therefore, no heparin should be used during dialysis. Anticoagulation could result in internal bleeding at the operative site. Blood pressure must also be defended. Any hypotensive episode during dialysis places the transplanted kidney at high risk of ischemia and necrosis. Finally, electrolyte imbalances must be resolved.

Advantage of having combined kidney/pancreas transplant

Quite commonly patients' renal failure is secondary to diabetes. In particular, type I diabetes causes renal failure in young persons. Therefore, a combined kidney/pancreatic transplant can alleviate both the renal failure as well as the hyperglycemia. The surgery is more complicated and the transplanted pancreas has a higher rate of rejection than the kidney alone. Moreover, the immunosuppressive regimen is far more complicated for the combined transplant. Yet, the potential benefits are great, particularly in young persons.

Duties of nephrology nurse caring for transplantation patient

The nephrology nurse who cares for the transplantation patient plays several important roles including the following:
- Education of the patient regarding transplantation
- Counseling the patient about transplantation
- Assisting patient with the pretransplant evaluation
- Providing dialysis treatments for those patients with transient loss of renal function due to acute tubular necrosis (ATN)

- Providing dialysis treatments for patients who have experienced permanent loss of a transplanted kidney
- Providing dialysis treatments for patients who are experiencing acute or chronic renal failure due to transplanted non-renal organs (heart or liver)

Immunosuppressant medications

The most common immunosuppressant classes are the following:
- Steroids—Blocks interleukin – 1 (a cytokine involved in the inflammatory cascade)
- Calcineurin inhibitors—Includes cyclosporine and tacrolimus block T cells reactions by blocking the signal calcineurin
- Antimetabolites—Include azathioprine and mycophenolate mofetil--act by blocking B cells
- Antilymphocytes—Include ATGAM and OKT3--block the actions of lymphocytes by targeting specific antigens on the lymphocytes
- Monoclonal antibodies—Include basiliximab and daclizumab-- are antibodies made to stop the actions of interleukin 2 (cytokine) and its binding with lymphocytes

Early signs and symptoms of rejection and infection for the post-transplant patient

It is important for the transplant patient to understand that up to 20% of patients will experience at least one episode of rejection. This does not mean, however, that they will lose their new kidney or that the kidney is not functioning the way it should. The patient should contact their transplant team if they experience a fever greater than 101 degrees, flu-like symptoms, decreased urine output, weight gain, or pain over the transplant site. Most often, blood work shows signs of rejection before the patient experiences many symptoms. Blood tests included complete blood counts, kidney function tests, electrolyte levels, and drug levels of the immunosuppressant medications. Regular kidney biopsies are also performed to test the kidney tissue itself for any markers that may reveal the early signs of rejection. There is extensive research being done to find more blood tests that check specific cell markers and other biomarkers that may indicate the kidney is showing signs of rejection. Other diagnostic tests that may be performed to visualize the mechanical function of the kidney include ultrasound, CT scan, or MRI.

Organ transplant process

Once the decision has been made to undergo a kidney transplant, the patient will work with a Clinical Transplant Coordinator. This person will be involved in coordinating all of the testing that is necessary to find a matching kidney, along with educating family members on the risks of organ donation. A Donor Coordinator is responsible for procuring and transporting the organ once a match has been found. Once the patient undergoes the surgical procedure to receive the new kidney, they will be in the ICU. The patient may need to continue dialysis until urine output is normal and the new kidney is functioning correctly. Fluids may be limited initially until the kidney is fully functioning. Immunosuppressant medications will be started and closely monitored to ensure the correct dosage is being received. The patient will receive consultation with a dietitian for any dietary guidelines they may need to follow. Physical therapy will also work with the patient to help with building strength. After discharge, there will be follow up appointments with the transplant surgeon to ensure the patient is healing appropriately and to be monitored for any signs of organ rejection.

Risks for infection and infection control techniques for post-transplant patients

Due to the immunosuppressant therapy the transplant patient must take, there is a greatly increased risk of infection. Pediatric patients tend to be at greater risk than adult patients. Bacterial infections are more common than viral infections, with UTIs and vascular access infections being most prevalent. Cytomegalovirus infections are the most common viral infection. Before the transplant surgery, the patient should receive any vaccines which they are lacking. If vaccines are requires post-surgery, inactivated vaccines should be given only. The risk of developing an infection from an active vaccine is greater than the benefit from receiving it post-transplant. The patient will be placed on prophylactic antibiotics to prevent UTI for up to one year following surgery. They may also be placed on antiviral therapy to prevent viral infection, usually for three months. Antifungal therapy may also be given depending upon the patient. The patient should be educated on their increased risk for infection and instructed in the importance of good handwashing. They should try to avoid others who they know are actively sick with an infectious disease. During epidemic levels of flu or other community illnesses, they should avoid large crowds to decrease their exposure.

Acute Therapies

Acute renal failure

Acute renal failure is defined as a 50% decrease in glomerular filtration rate (GFR). There are three broad categories where the causes of acute renal failure fall into:
- prerenal
- intrinsic
- postrenal

The pathophysiology of acute renal failure is poorly understood but particular attention must be given to those patients whom may require replacement therapy. Acute renal failure results in the buildup of nitrogenous waste, other toxins and metabolites (chiefly potassium, phosphorus, BUN, creatinine). The most concerning metabolite is potassium, which is a known cardiac toxin and can result in dangerous arrhythmias and death.

Common causes in children
The causes of acute renal failure in children are not that dissimilar from those causes seen in adults. These include:
- Prerenal azotemia from dehydration
- Sepsis
- Blood loss
- Nephrotoxic drugs such as aminoglycosides, nonsteriodal anti-inflammatory drugs (NDAIDS) and analgesics

However, the most common cause of acute renal failure in North American children is hemolytic uric syndrome, which can be seen with E.coli infections.

Indications for acute dialysis

The most common conditions in adults, infants and children that require acute dialysis are as follows:
- Symptomatic uremia, despite BUN and creatinine levels
- Pulmonary edema (a life-threatening complication of ARF), fluid overload, or acute myocardial infarction
- Hyperkalemia, when rapid reduction of plasma potassium level is indicated
- Acidosis, added sodium from IV sodium bicarbonate treatment may increase the chance of fluid volume overload
- Neurologic symptoms, toxic effects of uremia including headache, insomnia, lethargy, confusion, convulsions, and coma
- Drug overdose or poisoning, water-soluble drugs with low molecular weight (including ethanol, methanol, lithium and salicylates)

Drugs with high molecular weight (such as vancomycin and amphotericin B) or those that are protein bound (such as digoxin and acetylsalicylic acid), and lipid soluble drugs (for example, glutethimide) are not removed by dialysis.

Indications for urgent dialysis

The following are indications for urgent dialysis:
- A—<u>A</u>cidosis
- E—<u>E</u>lectrolyte imbalance (hyperkalemia is the most common)
- I—<u>I</u>ngestion of poisons or drugs
- O—Volume <u>O</u>verload
- U—<u>U</u>remic pericarditis or other uremic symptoms

Dialysis most affective in acute renal failure

Acute renal failure has a mortality rate of 40-50%. In order to prevent uremia due to the compromised kidney function, the patient will require renal replacement therapy, or dialysis. With acute renal failure, there are several choices for hemodialysis therapy. Intermittent hemodialysis, continuous renal replacement therapies, and hybrid therapies are available. With intermittent hemodialysis, dialysis is performed in scheduled, intermittent intervals. Continuous renal replacement therapy is used while the patient is inpatient in the ICU until the acute renal failure resolves and therapy is no longer needed. The hybrid therapies are categorized into sustained low-efficiency dialysis and extended-duration dialysis. The sustained low-efficiency dialysis provides continuous dialysis without the hemodynamic instability that can occur with continuous renal replacement therapy. Extended-duration dialysis is also a viable method of renal replacement therapy that helps to avoid the hemodynamic instability that can occur with continuous renal replacement therapy. Because of the avoidance of the hemodynamic instability that can occur with continuous dialysis, the hybrid therapies are preferred as a dialysis method in the acute renal failure patient.

Preventing acute decrease in glomerular filtration rates in patients with chronic kidney disease

The following is a list of interventions (as per KDOQI) which help **prevent** any acute insult to the kidneys and cause a decline in GFR:
- Volume depletion (can cause prerenal acute renal failure)
- Radiocontrast
- Antibiotics such as amphotericin and aminoglycosides
- Avoidance of non-steroidal anti-inflammatory drugs
- Avoidance of ace inhibitors and angiotensin receptor blockers (only if they acutely decrease the glomerular filtration rate; otherwise they are indicated for use in patients with chronic kidney disease)
- Preventing urinary tract obstructions
- Avoidance of certain chemotherapeutic agents such as tacrolimus and cyclosporine

Medications important in treatment of acute renal failure

In conjunction with dialysis, the following are medications that are important in the treatment of acute renal failure:
- Phosphate binders: With kidney failure, phosphates will accumulate in the body. Phosphate binders, such as calcium carbonate, will help to eliminate phosphates.
- Vitamin D: This is produced by the kidneys, so a supplemental form is necessary with kidney failure to ensure adequate bone strength.

- RBC Stimulating Agents: These replace the hormone erythropoietin, which is normally produced by the kidneys to stimulate red blood cell production.
- Iron: This is given if iron levels are low from the anemia that occurs with kidney failure.
- Stool softeners and/or laxatives: Constipation can occur due to decreased fluid intake.
- Vitamins: Vitamins B, C, and folic acid are removed during dialysis and supplements may be necessary to replace these.
- Antihypertensives: Especially ACE inhibitors, which are protective of the kidneys.
- Antibiotics: These may be necessary to treat infections at a peritoneal dialysis catheter site, such as with peritonitis.
- Heparin: This is frequently given to prevent fibrin threads from forming, which can block the dialysis catheter.
- Insulin: Diabetic patients who are undergoing peritoneal dialysis, may require adjustments in their insulin (or initiation of insulin if they have not used it before) due to the absorption of dextrose from the dialysate causing blood sugar levels to increase.

Patient education following acute renal failure and dialysis

The following are key elements in patient education that must be communicated to the patient following acute renal failure and dialysis:
- Following the physician's orders for any special diets or fluid restrictions. Keep a log of all foods and drinks consumed.
- Monitor urine output and record this at home.
- Weight yourself daily to evaluate for any fluid retention.
- Take your temperature every day and notify your physician's office if it should be above normal.
- Educate the patient on how to take their blood pressure at home. This should be monitored and recorded daily.
- Avoid friends or family members who are sick with an acute illness.
- Teach good handwashing techniques to avoid the spread of infection.
- Take medications exactly as prescribed.
- Keep any follow up appointments that have been scheduled with your physician.
- Contact the physician's office if you should develop symptoms of a UTI, fever >100 degrees, chills or sweats, gain or loss of more than 3 pounds in 24 hours, or swelling of the extremities.
- If the patient is discharged with a urinary catheter, they should monitor around the catheter insertion site for any redness or purulent drainage.
- Keep other medical conditions under adequate control, such as hypertension or diabetes, by following the medication instructions of your physician.

Practice Test

Practice Questions

Section Description: Jones Case Questions

Ben Jones, a 58-year-old patient with end-stage kidney disease (ESKD), has numerous complaints about his quality of life and is generally unhappy. Mr. Jones has had difficulties managing his treatment regimen.

1. Which of the following psychiatric disorders is most common in patients with ESKD?
    a. Anxiety.
    b. Dementia.
    c. Depression.
    d. Bipolar disorder.

2. Mr. Jones is screened with the Beck Depression Inventory and has a score of 20, suggesting
    a. no depression.
    b. mild depression.
    c. moderate depression.
    d. severe depression.

3. Mr. Jones participates in cognitive behavioral therapy to decrease depression, but his depression worsens, so the physician has prescribed a selective serotonin reuptake inhibitor (SSRI). For a patient with ESKD, the dosage of the SSRI should be
    a. reduced by two-thirds.
    b. increased by two-thirds.
    c. reduced by one-third.
    d. decreased by one-third.

4. Mr. Jones has not adhered to his diet plan, and the nurse is encouraging him to maintain a high-carbohydrate diet. The purpose of a high-carbohydrate diet for a patient with ESKD is to
    a. improve appetite.
    b. improve sense of well-being.
    c. spare protein for growth and healing.
    d. spare fat for growth and healing.

5. Mr. Jones' physical complaints may be associated with the MIA syndrome, which is commonly associated with ESKD. MIA refers to (1) malnutrition, (2) inflammation, and (3)
    a. anemia.
    b. agranulocytosis.
    c. angina.
    d. atherosclerosis.

Section Description: Maddox Case Questions

Jane Maddox is a 52-year-old woman who has started hemodialysis after both kidneys were removed because of bilateral renal cell carcinoma.

6. When teaching Ms. Maddox to manage fluid balance, the nurse advises the patient that a 1 kg (2.2 lb) increase in weight in 24 hours is approximately equivalent to fluid retention of
    a. 0.5 L.
    b. 1 L.
    c. 1.5 L.
    d. 2 L.

7. Ms. Maddox has been advised to avoid foods high in phosphorus. Foods that the patient should be advised to limit include
    a. fruits.
    b. vegetables.
    c. dairy products.
    d. grains.

8. Ms. Maddox has been prescribed sevelamer hydrochloride as a phosphate binder. The patient should be advised to take this medication
    a. 1 hour before meals.
    b. 2 hours after meals.
    c. first thing in the morning.
    d. with meals.

Section Description: Logan Case Questions

Artie Logan is a 40-year-old man with chronic kidney disease that has progressed from stage 2 to stage 3.

9. Chronic kidney disease is staged according to the patient's
    a. GFR.
    b. serum creatinine.
    c. BUN.
    d. urine albumin.

10. As chronic kidney disease progresses from stage 2 to stage 3, the focus of clinical intervention moves toward
    a. reducing risk and slowing progression.
    b. monitoring progression.
    c. preparing for dialysis.
    d. evaluating and treating complications.

Section Description: Carroll Case Questions

Estella Carroll, a 68-year-old woman with acute kidney injury and uremia, is receiving continuous renal therapy (CRRT) in the critical care unit.

11. Ms. Carroll is receiving continuous venovenous hemodialysis (CVVHD) because her severe uremia requires large volumes of fluid removal. What is the desirable mean arterial pressure (MAP) for optimal fluid removal and dialysis?
    a. At least 50 mm Hg.
    b. At least 60 mm Hg.
    c. At least 70 mm Hg.
    d. At least 80 mm Hg.

12. While Ms. Carroll is undergoing continuous renal replacement therapy, filter clotting occurs, slowing the ultrafiltration rate even after the nurse lowers the effluent container. The nurse should assess the system for
    a. disconnection of one of the lines.
    b. inappropriate dialysate.
    c. obstruction or inadequate heparinization.
    d. unsecured connections.

13. While Ms. Carroll is undergoing CVVHD with heparin used for anticoagulation, the nurse notes blood oozing from the catheter insertion site. Which of the following tests is indicated?
    a. Vitamin K level.
    b. Activated clotting time (ACT).
    c. Serum calcium.
    d. Hgb and Hct.

14. Ms. Carroll's condition stabilizes but she later becomes hypotensive, even though the lines are not disconnected and there is no blood leak. The nurse should suspect the cause is
    a. increased ultrafiltration rate
    b. sepsis.
    c. decreased ultrafiltration rate.
    d. myocardial infarction.

15. According to the CDC, to reduce the incidence of infection, Ms. Carroll's continuous renal replacement therapy (CRRT) catheter should be changed
    a. every 48 hours.
    b. every 5 days.
    c. once weekly.
    d. when clinically indicated.

16. According to the Kidney Disease: Improving Global Outcomes (KDIGO) acute kidney injury (AKI) guideline, CRRT is recommended over intermittent hemodialysis for patients with renal failure and
    a. heart failure.
    b. sepsis.
    c. cerebral edema.
    d. IV contrast administration.

Section Description: Mayer Case Questions

Sarah Mayer, a 26-year-old woman, develops hematuria, peripheral and pulmonary edema, hypertension, azotemia, and proteinuria, and is diagnosed with acute glomerulonephritis. The patient's BUN and serum creatinine levels are increased. The patient complains of headache, flank pain, and general malaise.

17. Ms. Mayer also presents with a malar rash, arthralgias, and oral lesions. Which disorder should be suspected as the precipitating factor for the acute glomerulonephritis?
    a. Rheumatoid arthritis.
    b. Systemic lupus erythematosus (SLE).
    c. Wegener granulomatosis.
    d. Renal cancer.

18. Based on these findings (including the malar rash, arthralgias, and oral lesions), in addition to a nephrologist, the patient may require consultation with a(n)
    a. oncologist.
    b. hematologist.
    c. immunologist.
    d. rheumatologist.

Section Description: Independent Questions, Group 1

19. Healthcare personnel caring for patients undergoing kidney transplantation should receive which of the following immunizations?
    a. Influenza (annual).
    b. Herpes zoster.
    c. Hepatitis C.
    d. DTaP.

20. The most common infection following kidney transplantation is
    a. abdominal.
    b. pulmonary.
    c. urinary tract.
    d. cardiovascular.

21. Twelve months after receiving a kidney transplant, a patient experiences reduced urinary output and increasing serum creatinine levels. Ultrasonography shows hydronephrosis is present. The most likely cause is
    a. renal artery stenosis.
    b. venous thrombosis.
    c. lymphocele.
    d. ureteral stenosis.

22. If a patient with a donor kidney develops sudden onset of hypertension 2 years after transplantation, the most likely cause is
    a. vascular thrombosis.
    b. ureteral obstruction.
    c. graft rejection.
    d. arterial stenosis.

23. Following kidney transplantation, a patient develops a large lymphocele between the bladder and the transplanted kidney. The treatment of choice is usually
    a. internal drainage into abdomen.
    b. sclerotherapy.
    c. instillation of fibrin glue.
    d. aspiration.

24. Kidney rejection within hours of transplantation is classified as
    a. accelerated.
    b. hyperacute.
    c. chronic.
    d. acute.

25. When OKT3 treatment is used for a severe acute kidney rejection episode, premedication usually begins with
    a. cyclosporine.
    b. azathioprine.
    c. methylprednisolone.
    d. fexofenadine.

26. According to the RIFLE criteria for acute kidney dysfunction, urinary output indicative of kidney failure is
    a. <0.5 mL/kg/h for 6 hours.
    b. <0.5 mL/kg/h for 12 hours.
    c. <0.3 mL/kg/h for 24 hours
    d. anuria for 6 hours.

27. Which of the following is an example of an intrarenal cause of AKI?
    a. Hemorrhage.
    b. Sepsis.
    c. Urethral obstruction.
    d. Tumor lysis syndrome.

28. Which of the following medications may result in tubular cell toxicity?
    a. Acetaminophen.
    b. Aminoglycosides.
    c. Diphenhydramine.
    d. Benzodiazepines.

29. If 200 patients are exposed to an airborne virus carried by a staff member over a 1-week period and 40 patients are infected, the attack rate is
    a. 5%.
    b. 10%.
    c. 20%.
    d. 40%.

30. If an infection involves a propagating source, the nurse would expect the infection to spread
    a. from a common source, such as the water supply.
    b. from person to person.
    c. through airborne means only.
    d. through contact only.

31. If 4 patients in a community of 2000 people are infected with methicillin-resistant *Staphylococcus aureus* (MRSA), this would be classified as a(n)
    a. epidemic.
    b. pandemic.
    c. outbreak.
    d. cluster.

32. The risk of disease occurring in a population (such as the number of people with kidney disease who develop a urinary tract infection) over a specified period of time (such as 1 year) is the
    a. incidence rate.
    b. prevalence rate.
    c. incidence density.
    d. attack rate.

Section Description: Aiken Case Questions

Drake Aiken, an 18-year-old man with ESKD resulting from IgA nephropathy, is to begin using continuous ambulatory peritoneal dialysis (CAPD) to control his condition.

33. When assisting a surgeon with stencil-based preoperative mapping for insertion of a peritoneal dialysis catheter, the nurse should initially position Mr. Aiken
    a. in any convenient position.
    b. standing.
    c. sitting.
    d. supine.

34. Prior to surgical placement of a catheter for peritoneal dialysis, the recommended antibiotic prophylaxis is generally
    a. aminoglycoside.
    b. vancomycin.
    c. sulfonamide.
    d. first-generation cephalosporin.

35. After a catheter is implanted, a culture of the catheter exit site is positive for *Staphylococcus aureus* but there is no erythema or purulent discharge. The most likely cause of the positive culture is
    a. peritonitis.
    b. lab error.
    c. colonization.
    d. specimen contamination.

36. Mr. Aiken receives instruction from the nurse about self-care and managing CAPD in the home environment. Which of the following is an acceptable method of warming dialysate for peritoneal dialysis in the home?
   a. Apply a heating pad.
   b. Immerse in warm water.
   c. Leave at room temperature for 3 hours.
   d. Hold under running warm water.

37. Once a dialysate bag is heated, the temperature can be assessed by
   a. Holding the bag against the wrist.
   b. Folding the bag over and enclosing an electronic thermometer.
   c. Inserting a thermometer into the tubing.
   d. Laying an electronic thermometer on top of the bag.

38. With CAPD, the number of exchanges that Mr. Aiken should expect to carry out in 24 hours is usually
   a. 2 to 3.
   b. 3 to 4.
   c. 4 to 5.
   d. 5 to 6.

39. In order to prevent gram-negative catheter-related infections, Mr. Aiken should avoid
   a. leaving the exit site uncovered.
   b. working outside in dusty conditions.
   c. taking hot showers.
   d. swimming in a lake.

40. With CAPD, the volume of dialysate retained in the peritoneal cavity at all times in adults, such as Mr. Aiken, is usually approximately
   a. ≤0.5 L.
   b. ≤1 L.
   c. ≤2 L.
   d. ≤3 L.

Section Description: Elmers Case Questions

> *Mary Jane Elmers is a 28-year-old woman on hemodialysis. Ms. Elmers is 3 months pregnant.*

41. Ms. Elmers' blood pressure is 160/100 mm Hg when she is euvolemic. An acceptable medication to treat hypertension in a pregnant patient on hemodialysis is
   a. labetalol.
   b. atenolol.
   c. ACE inhibitors.
   d. Angiotensin receptor blockers.

42. In order to increase the chance that Ms. Elmers will deliver a viable infant, ideally, she should be dialyzed
   a. on the same schedule as before pregnancy.
   b. 15 hours per week.
   c. <20 hours per week.
   d. >20 hours per week.

Section Description: Stephens Case Questions

Margaret Stephens is a 78-year-old woman with chronic kidney failure. She has remained fairly active despite the deterioration of her kidney function and heart failure.

43. Ms. Stephens has slightly impaired cognition because of decreased kidney function. The priority for patient education should be
   a. dietary and fluid restrictions.
   b. hygiene needs.
   c. pathophysiology of disease.
   d. exercise needs.

44. With chronic kidney failure, urine specific gravity usually ranges from
   a. 1.007 to 1.01.
   b. 1.01 to 1.015.
   c. 1.015 to 1.02
   d. 1.02 to 1.025.

45. If Ms. Stephen's cardiac output decreases, resulting in arterial hypoperfusion with reduced blood flow to the kidneys, the nurse expects lab results to show
   a. increased BUN.
   b. decreased BUN.
   c. increased GFR.
   d. stable BUN and decreased GFR.

46. In elderly patients, such as Ms. Stephens, with kidney failure, the first signs of various types of infection may be
   a. rash and somnolence.
   b. fever and confusion.
   c. fever and incontinence.
   d. confusion and incontinence.

47. Prior to a serum creatinine test, Ms. Stephens should be advised to
   a. avoid excessive exercise.
   b. avoid food and fluids for 12 hours.
   c. drink 3 to 4 glasses of water.
   d. avoid fluids for 6 hours.

48. With kidney disease, decreased urine specific gravity may result from
    a. volume excess.
    b. glycosuria.
    c. volume deficit.
    d. proteinuria.

Section Description: Independent Questions, Group 2

49. The primary preventive measure to avoid contrast-induced nephrotoxic injury for a patient who must receive IV radiopaque contrast material despite chronic kidney dysfunction is
    a. IV sodium bicarbonate.
    b. oral N-acetylcysteine.
    c. IV normal saline.
    d. IV fenoldopam.

50. Which of the following ethnic groups is most at risk for development of kidney failure?
    a. Caucasians.
    b. Hispanic Americans.
    c. Asians.
    d. African Americans.

51. If the goal is to utilize a simple display of data to show patients and staff progress in decreasing infections in patients with kidney disease each month over the past year, the best display type is likely a
    a. bar graph.
    b. line graph.
    c. pie graph.
    d. histogram.

52. Which of the following agencies is responsible for the safety of the nation's blood supply and sets standards for blood collection, testing, and distribution?
    a. OSHA.
    b. CDC.
    c. FDA.
    d. CMS.

53. If a patient with chronic kidney failure develops pyelonephritis, the antibiotic of choice is generally a(n)
    a. cephalosporin.
    b. aminoglycoside.
    c. penicillin.
    d. fluoroquinolone.

54. The primary complication from recurrent pyelonephritis is
    a. scarring.
    b. sepsis.
    c. pericarditis.
    d. hypertension.

55. Following a percutaneous kidney biopsy for diagnostic purposes, the most common complication is
   a. severe pain.
   b. arteriovenous fistula.
   c. hematuria.
   d. hematoma.

56. With the renin-angiotensin-aldosterone system (RAAS), in response to decreased renal blood flow and decreased pressure in the glomerulus,
   a. renin is decreased.
   b. renin is released.
   c. aldosterone is released.
   d. Na reabsorption decreases.

57. Nephrotic syndrome is characterized by
   a. marked proteinuria.
   b. hematuria.
   c. hypertension.
   d. dehydration.

58. Patients may be advised to fast for at least 4 hours prior to a CT of the kidney with IV iodinated contrast because
   a. fasting improves images.
   b. physician preference only.
   c. patients may experience nausea and vomiting.
   d. some foods may interact with the contrast material.

59. Which of the following are the primary causes of nephrosclerosis?
   a. Hypertension and diabetes.
   b. Hypertension and hepatitis B.
   c. Hypertension and HIV.
   d. Hypertension and kidney trauma.

60. Shortly after emergency department admission for post-infectious acute glomerulonephritis, a patient develops altered mental status. The most likely cause of this complication is
   a. anemia.
   b. dehydration.
   c. hypertensive encephalopathy.
   d. hyponatremia.

61. Prerenal kidney failure may result from
   a. nephrotoxic agents.
   b. urinary tract obstruction.
   c. prolonged renal ischemia.
   d. volume depletion.

62. Which of the following laboratory findings is characteristic of acute prerenal kidney failure?
    a. Na <20 mEq/L.
    b. Na >20 mEq/L.
    c. Na <40 mEq/L.
    d. Na >40 mEq/L.

63. The obligatory urinary output that is needed to filter normal metabolic waste products and remove them from the body is about
    a. 300 mL.
    b. 500 mL.
    c. 700 mL.
    d. 800 mL.

64. Which of the following medications is nephrotoxic and should have baseline and follow-up BUN and serum creatinine monitored during administration?
    a. Metoprolol.
    b. Acetaminophen.
    c. Calcitriol.
    d. Vancomycin.

65. If a patient with kidney failure has an order for a sodium polystyrene sulfonate (Kayexalate) retention enema, the nurse expects that the patient is being treated for
    a. hypokalemia.
    b. hyperkalemia.
    c. hypophosphatemia.
    d. hyperphosphatemia.

66. A patient with acute kidney failure is stabilizing and seems alert and responsive, but the nurse notes that the patient needs to have explanations for treatments and procedures repeated many times. The most likely reason is
    a. anemia.
    b. encephalopathy.
    c. fatigue.
    d. anxiety.

67. According to KDIGO acute kidney injury guideline, CRRT for patients with acute kidney injury should deliver effluent volume of
    a. 15 to 20 mL/h.
    b. 20 to 25 mL/h.
    c. 25 to 30 mL/h.
    d. 30 to 35 mL/h.

68. A new nurse in the critical care unit is unfamiliar with CRRT equipment being used and works very slowly because of the need to check procedures, which increases the workload of other staff members. The best solution is to
    a. complain to the director.
    b. advise the new nurse to take materials home to study.
    c. allow the new nurse all the time needed to learn.
    d. offer to assist and mentor the new nurse.

69. Which of the following forms of CRRT does not provide fluid replacement?
    a. Continuous venovenous hemodiafiltration (CVVHDF).
    b. Continuous venovenous hemodialysis (CVVHD).
    c. Continuous venovenous hemofiltration (CVVH).
    d. Slow continuous ultrafiltration (SCUF).

Section Description: Mayweather Case Questions

Dan Mayweather is a 48-year-old man who has received peritoneal dialysis for 5 years but has recently changed to in-center hemodialysis. Mr. Mayweather is preparing to switch to home hemodialysis.

70. Mr. Mayweather has developed pain and stiffness in the joints. The most likely cause is
    a. osteoarthritis.
    b. rheumatoid arthritis.
    c. amyloidosis.
    d. gout.

71. Mr. Mayweather complains of severe itching during and after hemodialysis despite taking a phosphate binder. Which medication is commonly prescribed to help relieve the itching?
    a. Prednisone.
    b. Calcitriol.
    c. Diazepam.
    d. Diphenhydramine.

72. A primary advantage of home hemodialysis is
    a. more frequent treatments.
    b. lower risk of infection.
    c. lower cost.
    d. longer fistula survival.

73. Mr. Mayweather has opted to have a buttonhole technique for hemodialysis. Which of the following is the most important factor for creation of a buttonhole tract for hemodialysis?
    a. The originator should document the exact site and angle of needle insertion.
    b. A team of at least 2 cannulators should alternate treatments until the tunnel is established.
    c. The patient should do all cannulations until the tunnel is established.
    d. The same cannulator should do treatments until the tunnel is established.

74. The nurse is teaching Mr. Mayweather about aseptic techniques. If using a combination chlorhexidine gluconate and alcohol skin prep (such as ChloraPrep) before cannulation, how much skin contact time is required?
    a. 15 seconds.
    b. 30 seconds.
    c. 60 seconds.
    d. 3 minutes.

75. Mr. Mayweather has buttonhole tracks for access and is being taught to carry out treatments with the assistance of his wife. After the area is cleansed and prepped for treatment, what is the next step?
   a. Insert sharp needles into the tracts.
   b. Insert blunt needles into the tracts.
   c. Use a scab picker/aseptic tweezers to remove the scabs.
   d. Use the treatment needle to remove the scabs.

76. With buttonhole tracks, Mr. Mayweather should be taught to apply pressure as the needles are removed and then for
   a. 1 to 2 minutes.
   b. 5 to 10 minutes.
   c. 10 to 20 minutes.
   d. 20 to 30 minutes.

77. If Mr. Mayweather's buttonhole access frequently has long clots that are very difficult to remove, the most likely reason is
   a. subclinical infection.
   b. use of improper needle.
   c. failure to use 2-finger hold for needle removal.
   d. failure to adequately remove previous clot before cannulation.

78. With buttonhole access sites, what should Mr. Mayweather do to prevent "hubbing?"
   a. Leave 1/16th to 1/8th inch of the needle exposed.
   b. Insert the needle just to the hub.
   c. Use a sharp needle to remove scabs.
   d. Use a long catheter so the hub is not close to the site.

79. The amount of dialysis that Mr. Mayweather is prescribed is based on the removal of
   a. urea.
   b. creatinine.
   c. potassium.
   d. albumin.

80. Mr. Mayweather complains that he frequently experiences muscle cramping during hemodialysis. The most common predisposing factor for muscle cramping during hemodialysis is
   a. electrolyte imbalance.
   b. low ultrafiltration rate.
   c. high sodium dialysis solution.
   d. hypotension.

81. The nurse is teaching Mr. Mayweather about complications that may arise during hemodialysis. Which of the following is an indication that there is clotting in the extracorporeal circuit?
   a. Very light bright blood.
   b. White streaks in the dialyzer.
   c. Teetering blood in the arterial line segment.
   d. Foaming and clots in drip chamber.

82. The nurse advises Mr. Mayweather that foam in the venous blood line of a dialyzer may indicate
   a. normal finding.
   b. sepsis.
   c. air embolism.
   d. too rapid blood flow rate.

Section Description: Bell Case Questions

Mary Bell is a 56-year-old woman scheduled for a kidney transplant because of autosomal dominant polycystic kidney disease. For the previous 4 years, she has been treated with hemodialysis.

83. Ms. Bell's partner has volunteered to be a living donor. The primary concern when evaluating the donor is
   a. general health.
   b. insurance coverage.
   c. blood type.
   d. psychological status.

84. Which of the following pre-transplant screenings is recommended for adult recipients of a donor kidney?
   a. Urinalysis.
   b. Varicella-zoster virus antibody.
   c. West Nile virus.
   d. *Trypanosoma cruzi.*

85. Ms. Bell's BMI is 29 kg/m². Increased morbidity and mortality after kidney transplant is associated with BMI of
   a. >26 kg/m2.
   b. >28 kg/m2.
   c. >30 kg/m2.
   d. >40 kg/m2.

86. Ms. Bell undergoes a psychiatric evaluation as part of screening procedures. Which of the following information gleaned during a psychiatric consultation is most likely to be a contraindication for kidney transplant?
   a. History of depression.
   b. History of nonadherence to treatment regimen.
   c. History of substance abuse.
   d. History of unemployment.

87. Following kidney transplantation, IV fluids are administered for maintenance and for replacement of lost fluids. How much insensible loss is anticipated per hour?
   a. 10 mL.
   b. 30 mL.
   c. 45 mL.
   d. 60 mL.

88. In the immediate postoperative period after kidney transplantation, the physician should be notified if urinary output is
   a. <50 mL for 1 hour.
   b. >500 mL for 1 hour.
   c. >150 mL/h for 4 hours.
   d. <60 mL/h for 2 consecutive hours.

89. Following kidney transplantation, Ms. Bell develops a small bladder leak. Initial treatment usually includes
   a. surgical repair of leak.
   b. Foley catheter and decompression.
   c. cystectomy.
   d. instillation of antibiotic solution.

90. Ms. Bell must take immunosuppressive agents to prevent transplant rejection. Which of the following immunosuppressive agents used to prevent kidney rejection after transplantation is the most nephrotoxic?
   a. Cyclosporine.
   b. Azathioprine.
   c. Methylprednisolone.
   d. Mycophenolate mofetil.

91. When Ms. Bell is discharged after kidney transplantation, the nurse should ensure the patient understands that the primary measures to determine the health of the kidney are
   a. serum creatinine and urinary output.
   b. BUN and urinary output.
   c. BUN and serum creatinine.
   d. urinary output and blood pressure.

92. Ms. Bell undergoes periodic core needle biopsies to assess the condition of the kidney. The most common complication associated with core needle biopsy of a transplanted kidney is
   a. arteriovenous fistula.
   b. ureteral obstruction.
   c. bleeding/hematuria.
   d. infection.

93. Six months after transplantation, Ms. Bell exhibits signs of depression. The medicine of choice to treat depression after kidney transplantation is usually
   a. an SSRI.
   b. an MAO inhibitor.
   c. a tricyclic antidepressant.
   d. St. John's wort.

Section Description: Independent Questions, Group 3

94. The greatest risk of bacteremia is associated with which type of vascular access?
   a. Primary arteriovenous fistula.
   b. Arteriovenous graft (biologic).
   c. Dialysis catheter.
   d. Arteriovenous graft (prosthetic).

95. Which of the following antiseptics used for skin prep for a fistula site has the broadest spectrum antibacterial activity?
    a. Povidone iodine.
    b. Isopropyl alcohol 70%.
    c. Chlorhexidine gluconate 2%.
    d. Hydrogen peroxide.

96. If a patient develops an infection of a primary arteriovenous (AV) fistula and requires more than 6 weeks of antibiotic treatment, which of the following conditions should be expected?
    a. Subacute endocarditis.
    b. Sepsis.
    c. Pericarditis.
    d. Encephalitis.

97. While a patient is undergoing hemodialysis, chloramine testing should be conducted every
    a. hour.
    b. 2 hours.
    c. 4 hours.
    d. 5 hours.

98. The last component of the water processing system before the distribution loop should be a(n)
    a. ultrafilter.
    b. ultraviolet light.
    c. reverse osmosis device.
    d. deionizer.

99. Fluoride contamination of water used for hemodialysis may result in
    a. hemolysis.
    b. ventricular fibrillation.
    c. anemia.
    d. encephalopathy.

100. A patient has had a prosthetic arteriovenous graft implanted. Maturation usually takes
    a. 1 to 3 weeks.
    b. 3 to 6 weeks.
    c. 1 to 2 months.
    d. 2 to 4 month.

101. Which of the following contaminants of water used for dialysis may result in dialysis dementia?
    a. Zinc.
    b. Chloramine.
    c. Copper.
    d. Aluminum.

102. If a hemodialysis patient presents with shaking chills, high fever, myalgia, hypotension, nausea, and vomiting, the most likely causative agent is
   a. gram-negative bacteria.
   b. gram-positive bacteria.
   c. endotoxin.
   d. nontubercular *Mycobacterium*.

103. If a patient with acute tubular necrosis is receiving hemodialysis, which phase of the disease may be obscured?
   a. Oliguria/Anuria.
   b. Diuresis.
   c. Recovery.
   d. Onset.

104. A postmenopausal hemodialysis patient complains of dyspareunia. The most effective treatment is likely
   a. vaginal lubricant.
   b. sustained-release intravaginal estrogen ring.
   c. psychological counseling.
   d. conjugated estrogen cream.

105. For a hemodialysis cannulation with a blood flow rate of less than 300 mL/min, which of the following needle gauge sizes is usually recommended?
   a. 14.
   b. 15.
   c. 16.
   d. 17.

106. The use of topical anesthetics, such as EMLA, to reduce discomfort during cannulation is contraindicated with
   a. buttonhole sites.
   b. AV fistulas.
   c. AV grafts.
   d. all hemodialysis patients.

107. If a dialysis center is utilizing Continuous Quality Improvement methods, the question that the nurse should continually ask is
   a. "How can the center do things better?"
   b. "How can I avoid errors?"
   c. "How can the center be more cost effective?"
   d. "What is the staff doing right?"

108. Early symptoms of disequilibrium syndrome associated with long-term hemodialysis include
   a. seizures and coma.
   b. hypertension and tachycardia.
   c. headache, nausea, and vomiting.
   d. headache and respiratory distress.

109. An 80-year-old patient with ESKD is a candidate for hemodialysis, but the patient refuses treatment, stating that death is preferable to the loss of independence and continued illness. The nurse should
    a. respect the patient's decision.
    b. suggest the patient see a psychiatrist.
    c. try to convince the patient of the benefits of hemodialysis.
    d. remind the patient that he will die soon without treatment.

110. If a patient with diabetes mellitus at high risk for kidney disease is negative for macroscopic protein with dipstick testing, the nurse expects the next step to be
    a. doing dipstick testing at all follow-up visits.
    b. assuming the patient is not at risk.
    c. testing for microalbuminuria.
    d. serum creatinine.

111. The nurse is teaching a hemodialysis patient who still urinates to manage fluid intake with a base of 1000 mL intake per day. If the patient urinates 500 mL in a 24-hour period, how much fluid is the patient allowed the following day?
    a. 1500 mL.
    b. 1000 mL.
    c. 1250 mL.
    d. 1300 mL.

112. If a patient who usually drinks 2 cups of caffeinated coffee each morning has headaches during hemodialysis, the patient should be advised to
    a. stop drinking coffee altogether.
    b. drink a cup of strong coffee with treatment.
    c. skip coffee the morning of the treatment.
    d. transition to decaffeinated beverages.

113. Which of the following agencies/organizations sets the minimally adequate target spKt/V as a clinical performance measure for all outpatient dialysis centers in the United States?
    a. FDA.
    b. OSHA.
    c. CDC.
    d. CMS.

114. The electronic event reporting documentation form for the dialysis center is lengthy and time-consuming and not always applicable to the center, causing staff members to avoid making reports of near-misses despite guidelines that require them to do so. The best solution is to
    a. keep alternate records for near misses.
    b. assign a staff person to ensure all events are recorded.
    c. identify those elements of the form that require modification.
    d. complain to the administration that the form is too time-consuming.

115. For which of the following sleep disorders should all hemodialysis patients be screened?
    a. Insomnia.
    b. Restless legs syndrome (RLS).
    c. Obstructive sleep apnea.
    d. Periodic limb movements in sleep (PLMS).

116. If a sentinel event, such as death resulting from exsanguination, occurs, the initial response must include
   a. conducting a root cause analysis.
   b. firing the staff involved.
   c. determining who was to blame.
   d. consulting attorneys.

117. A patient on hemodialysis suffered a myocardial infarction (MI) and remains weak. The patient has not resumed any exercise because of fear of another MI. The patient may benefit the most from a referral to a
   a. psychiatrist.
   b. support group.
   c. cardiac rehabilitation program.
   d. physical therapist.

Section Description: Evans Case Questions

> *Sally Evans, a 48-year-old woman, has been using peritoneal dialysis for the past year. Swabs of her nares indicate that she is colonized with Staphylococcus aureus.*

118. Which of the following may be indicated to prevent exit-site infections for Ms. Evans while she is undergoing peritoneal dialysis?
   a. Application of hydrogen peroxide to exit site.
   b. Application of transparent dressing over exit site.
   c. Application of mupirocin cream to exit site.
   d. Application of clindamycin gel to exit site.

119. Ms. Evans notes that the dialysis effluent is cloudy. For a patient undergoing peritoneal dialysis, when sending a sample of cloudy dialysate for culture and sensitivities, what is the minimal sample size?
   a. 5 mL.
   b. 10 mL.
   c. 20 mL.
   d. 30 mL.

120. Ms. Evans develops tenderness about the catheter site and purulent discharge. Which of the following additional signs/symptoms are included in the minimal diagnostic criteria for peritonitis?
   a. Fever and dialysate WBC count of 50 cells/mm3 and 25 PMN leukocytes.
   b. Cloudy dialysate and dialysate WBC count of 50 cells/mm3 and 25 PMN leukocytes.
   c. Abdominal pain and dialysate WBC count of 50 cells/mm3 and 30 PMN leukocytes.
   d. Abdominal pain and dialysate WBC count of >100 cells/mm3 and 50 PMN leukocytes.

121. Ms. Evans is diagnosed with peritonitis. The most common pathogen isolated from patients with peritoneal dialysis–associated peritonitis is
   a. coagulase-negative *Staphylococcus.*
   b. *Staphylococcus aureus.*
   c. *Pseudomonas aeruginosa.*
   d. Enterobacteriaceae.

122. Ms. Evans is being treated for peritonitis. If fibrinous clots are visible in the dialysis effluent, the treatment of choice is
   a. heparin.
   b. warfarin.
   c. dabigatran.
   d. apixaban.

Section Description: Walker Case Questions

Stephanie Walker is a 20-year-old college student with chronic kidney disease.

123. Ms. Walker has required frequent hospitalizations because of her nonadherence to the treatment plan. The best approach to take with the patient is to
   a. point out how the patient has caused the hospitalizations.
   b. ask the patient how the nurse can help her better manage her condition.
   c. suggest that the patient needs to act in a more mature manner.
   d. advise the patient that she may benefit from psychological counseling.

124. Ms. Walker questions whether she will be able to have children. A patient of childbearing age with which of the following kidney diseases may be referred to a genetics counselor when considering pregnancy?
   a. Chronic pyelonephritis.
   b. Polycystic kidney disease (PKD).
   c. Glomerulonephritis.
   d. Nephrotic syndrome.

125. The nurse feels a special friendship toward Ms. Walker, who reminds the nurse of a close family member. The nurse should deal with this by
   a. acknowledging the feeling.
   b. asking for reassignment.
   c. avoiding the patient when possible.
   d. spending extra time with the patient.

Section Description: Garcia Case Questions

Jose Garcia is a 64-year-old man on hemodialysis because of kidney failure related to type 2 diabetes mellitus.

126. Mr. Garcia is receiving hemodialysis with 17-gauge needles and has a blood flow rate of 450 mL/min. He complains of sudden onset of chest tightness, back pain, and dyspnea, and the nurse notes a reddening of skin color and blood in the venous line appearing port-wine in color. Which complication is most likely?
   a. Disequilibrium syndrome.
   b. Hemolysis.
   c. Air embolism.
   d. Cardiac tamponade.

127. Based on Mr. Garcia's symptoms, the immediate action should be to
   a. slow the blood flow rate to <400 mL/min.
   b. administer normal saline.
   c. stop the blood pump and clamp the blood lines.
   d. monitor electrolytes.

128. For which electrolyte imbalance should Mr. Garcia be monitored?
   a. Hyperkalemia.
   b. Hypokalemia.
   c. Hypophosphatemia.
   d. Hyperphosphatemia.

129. According to NKF KDOQI guidelines, patients, such as Mr. Garcia, receiving hemodialysis should receive treatment with an active vitamin D sterol (such as calcitriol) when parathyroid hormone (PTH) levels are
   a. >150 pg/mL.
   b. >200 pg/mL.
   c. >300 pg/mL.
   d. >400 pg/mL.

130. After initiation of calcitriol treatment for elevated PTH level, Mr. Garcia's calcium level is 10.5 mg/dL. The appropriate response is to
   a. increase calcitriol dose by 25%.
   b. decrease calcitriol dose by 25%.
   c. decrease calcitriol dose by 50%.
   d. hold the calcitriol.

131. Which of the following statements by Mr. Garcia most suggests that the patient may need a referral for psychological counseling?
   a. "I hate having to come for treatments 3 times a week."
   b. "It's hard for me to keep up at work."
   c. "Some days I wish I didn't even wake up."
   d. "Living with kidney failure is pretty miserable at times."

Section Description: Independent Questions, 3

132. An 18-year-old female patient with continuous ambulatory peritoneal dialysis (CAPD) has become increasingly withdrawn and is reluctant to be seen in public unless wearing a large coat. The patient is most likely experiencing
   a. body image disturbance.
   b. activity intolerance.
   c. ineffective thermoregulation.
   d. ineffective coping.

133. Considering the peritoneal equilibrium test (PET), patients in which of the following transporter categories would be expected to have the highest 4-hour dialysate to plasma creatinine, urea, and sodium (D/PCr, PUr, and PNa) values?
   a. Low transporters.
   b. Low-average transporters.
   c. High-average transporters.
   d. High transporters.

134. A patient with CAPD has decreased effluent volumes of dialysate and increased weight gain without peripheral edema. Physical examination shows an asymmetric protuberant abdomen. The most likely cause is
   a. abdominal wall leak.
   b. peri-catheter leak.
   c. hydrothorax.
   d. peritonitis.

135. A patient with CAPD has resorted to increasingly frequent use of more hypertonic glucose dialysate in order to prevent fluid overload and achieve target weight. The initial intervention should be to
   a. decrease sodium and fluid intake.
   b. increase sodium intake and decrease fluid intake.
   c. further increase hypertonicity.
   d. decrease hypertonicity.

136. Which of the following diffuses from peritoneal capillary blood into peritoneal fluid during peritoneal dialysis?
   a. Glucose.
   b. Albumin.
   c. Bicarbonate.
   d. Potassium.

137. Amino acid–based solution for peritoneal dialysis is indicated for
   a. all patients.
   b. nutritionally compromised patients.
   c. diabetic patients.
   d. pregnant patients.

138. An upper chest presternal exit site for peritoneal dialysis may be indicated for
   a. patients wearing belt line above umbilicus.
   b. patients who are morbidly obese.
   c. younger patients.
   d. wheelchair-bound patients.

139. Mixing which of the following antibiotics with penicillin in the same dialysis solution bag is contraindicated?
   a. Vancomycin.
   b. Cefazolin.
   c. Ceftazidime.
   d. Gentamicin.

140. For what duration is vancomycin stable in dialysate stored at room temperature?
   a. 4 days.
   b. 7 days.
   c. 14 days.
   d. 28 days.

141. A patient with peritoneal dialysis is receiving intraperitoneal (IP) fluconazole for fungal peritonitis and begins to experience hallucinations and exhibit paranoid behavior. The nurse should suspect
   a. psychotic break.
   b. overdose.
   c. allergic response.
   d. adverse effect.

142. A patient on peritoneal dialysis tells the nurse that one of the employees at the patient's company has offered to give him a kidney in exchange for $100,000. The nurse should advise the patient that
   a. the employee may not be a match.
   b. it is illegal to buy or sell an organ.
   c. the employee should come for compatibility testing.
   d. the patient should keep the financial arrangement secret.

Section Description: Woods Case Questions

   Tamara Woods is a 78-year-old female who is critically ill in the hospital ICU after a motor vehicle accident. She has developed acute kidney injury (AKI).

143. The most common cause of acute kidney injury in critically ill patients is
   a. older age.
   b. heart failure.
   c. pneumonia.
   d. sepsis.

144. Ms. Woods' ECG telemetry shows peaked T waves and widening of the QRS interval. These changes may be indicative of
   a. hyperkalemia.
   b. hypokalemia
   c. hypernatremia.
   d. hyponatremia.

145. If Ms. Woods has increasing peripheral edema and pulmonary congestion with decreased urinary output, the medication of choice is likely
   a. a thiazide diuretic.
   b. an osmotic diuretic.
   c. a loop diuretic.
   d. a potassium-sparing diuretic.

146. Ms. Woods becomes anuric despite treatment, and her potassium level rapidly increases from 4.5 to 6 mmol/L. The most likely temporary emergent treatment is
   a. loop diuretic.
   b. insulin and glucose.
   c. sodium polystyrene sulfonate.
   d. intravenous normal saline.

147. If Ms. Woods' serum creatinine increases from 0.75 to 1.5 mg/dL, what effect on the GFR does the nurse expect?
   a. Increase 50%.
   b. Decrease 50%.
   c. Increase 25%.
   d. Decrease 25%.

Section Description: Washington Case Questions

> *Jasper Washington is a 56-year-old man with type 2 diabetes mellitus. Mr. Washington is newly diagnosed with ESKD and in need of peritoneal dialysis.*

148. When instructing Mr. Washington in the use of a preattached double bag system for peritoneal dialysis, he should be advised to flush how much dialysate from the fill bag to the drainage bag before filling the peritoneal cavity?
   a. 25 mL.
   b. 50 mL.
   c. 75 mL.
   d. 100 mL.

149. When teaching Mr. Washington about dialysate, the nurse should understand that the primary advantage of a 2-compartment peritoneal dialysis solution bag is to
   a. allow delivery at normal pH.
   b. maintain pH at 5.5.
   c. decrease risk of infection.
   d. allow 2 different solutions to be instilled sequentially.

150. The nurse teaches Mr. Washington that the 3 transport processes that occur during the course of peritoneal dialysis are (1) diffusion, (2) ultrafiltration, and (3)
   a. absorption.
   b. radiation.
   c. transference.
   d. conduction.

Section Description: Lee Case Questions

> *Darlene Lee, a 38-year-old woman with ESKD, is scheduled to begin hemodialysis and has had an AV fistula created.*

151. A week after Ms. Lee has an AV fistula created in the lower arm, the patient is referred to physical therapy for exercises to help mature the fistula. Exercises that the patient is advised to do likely include
    a. swinging the arm in circles.
    b. bicep curls.
    c. hammer curls.
    d. ball squeezes.

152. During the first week of treatment with a new AV fistula, the initial needle size and blood flow rate are usually
    a. 14-gauge needle and blood flow of 200 to 250 mL/min.
    b. 16-gauge needle and blood flow of 250 to 300 mL/min.
    c. 17-gauge needle and blood flow of 200 to 250 mL/min.
    d. 17-gauge needle and blood flow of 300 to 350 mL/min.

153. With an AV fistula, cannulation should be done at an angle of
    a. 15° to 25°.
    b. 25° to 35°.
    c. 45°.
    d. 45° to 60°.

154. According to one element of the "Rule of 6s," an AV fistula is considered successful if it
    a. is 6 inches long.
    b. is 0.06 cm below the skin surface.
    c. has a 60 mL/min blood flow rate.
    d. is 0.6 cm wide.

155. If an infection occurs in an arteriovenous graft, Ms. Lee is at increased risk of
    a. hemorrhage.
    b. dialysis dementia.
    c. fluoride intoxication.
    d. hyperglycemia.

Case Description: Shaw Case Questions

> *Mr. Stanley Shaw is a 64-year-old man who has been using automated peritoneal dialysis (APD) for the past 2 years.*

156. For a patient such as Mr. Shaw receiving APD with most dialysis occurring during the night, the best time to take a plasma sample to determine the urea level is
    a. at bedtime.
    b. on arising.
    c. noon.
    d. mid-afternoon.

157. With APD, icodextrin may be used rather than glucose solution for
    a. all short daytime dwells.
    b. 1 long day dwell.
    c. long nocturnal dwell.
    d. all dwells, day and night.

158. With APD, how many nighttime hours would Mr. Shaw spend cycling?
    a. 4 to 6.
    b. 6 to 8.
    c. 8 to 10.
    d. 10 to 12.

Section Description: Rule Case Questions

James Rule is a 70-year-old patient who developed hemolytic uremic syndrome (HUS) as the result of an Escherichia coli (O157:H7) infection.

159. HUS is characterized by the triad of (1) acute renal failure, (2) microangiopathic hemolytic anemia, and (3)
    a. thrombocytosis.
    b. thrombocytopenia.
    c. leukocytosis.
    d. leukopenia.

160. Initial therapy for HUS usually includes
    a. broad-spectrum antibiotics.
    b. antidiarrheal agents.
    c. antiplatelet agents.
    d. intravenous fluids.

161. With HUS, the part of the kidney that is damaged is the
    a. glomeruli.
    b. loop of Henle.
    c. distal tubules.
    d. papillae.

Section Description: Branch Case Study

Thomas Branch is a 60-year old hospitalized man, newly diagnosed with kidney failure and started on CAPD.

162. Mr. Branch has little income, inadequate insurance, and little social support. The best initial referral is to
    a. Medicaid.
    b. a social worker.
    c. a home health agency.
    d. a free clinic.

163. When teaching Mr. Branch to manage CAPD, the nurse is concerned that he may lack the manual dexterity needed to manage the procedure. The best professional to assess this is a(n)
    a. occupational therapist.
    b. rehabilitation specialist.
    c. home health nurse.
    d. physical therapist.

164. Which of the following statements by Mr. Branch when he is undergoing peritoneal dialysis indicates the need for referral to a nutritionist?
    a. "I should have 30 to 40 grams of fiber daily."
    b. "I can have all of the salt and salty foods I want in my diet."
    c. "I should choose soft cheese over hard."
    d. "I drink ginger ale instead of cola."

165. Mr. Branch is concerned about losing employment because of the inability to carry out all aspects of the job due to physical limitations. The best initial solution for the patient is likely to
    a. apply for disability through Social Security.
    b. ask for accommodations per the ADA.
    c. look for other employment.
    d. retrain for other types of employment.

166. If Mr. Branch frequently exhibits denial regarding physical decline but adheres closely to treatment regimens and remains cheerful, the best response to this patient's denial is to
    a. refer the patient for psychological counseling.
    b. allow patient to use denial.
    c. assist the patient to develop a more realistic attitude.
    d. point out where the patient is in error.

Section Description: Anders Case Questions

Marian Anders, a 72-year-old woman with type 2 diabetes mellitus, has chronic kidney disease.

167. A patient with diabetes mellitus and chronic kidney disease should generally have a target HbA_{1c} of
    a. <5%.
    b. <6%.
    c. <7%.
    d. <8%.

168. In a diabetic patient with chronic kidney disease, glycosuria
    a. is a good estimation of hyperglycemia.
    b. may occur without hyperglycemia.
    c. is unreliable as an estimation of hyperglycemia.
    d. is almost always absent.

169. When teaching a patient with chronic kidney disease about dietary restrictions, the nurse should generally advise the patient to limit daily protein intake to
   a. 0.6 g/kg.
   b. 0.8 g/kg.
   c. 1 g/kg.
   d. 2 g/kg.

170. Patients such as Ms. Anders with chronic kidney disease often develop which type of anemia because of decreased production of erythropoietin?
   a. Microcytic, hypochromic.
   b. Microcytic, normochromic.
   c. Normocytic, normochromic.
   d. Normocytic, hypochromic.

171. Mrs. Anders' hemoglobin is 11 g/d. According to KDIGO guidelines, treatment for chronic kidney disease with an erythropoiesis-stimulating agent should not be initiated until the hemoglobin level falls to
   a. <9 g/dL.
   b. <10 g/dL.
   c. <11 g/dL.
   d. <12 g/dL.

172. As chronic kidney disease progresses, which endocrinologic change can result in higher risk of fractures?
   a. Hypothyroidism.
   b. Hyperthyroidism.
   c. Hyperparathyroidism.
   d. Hypoparathyroidism.

173. Kidney failure is generally considered inevitable when loss of kidney function reaches
   a. 30% to 40%.
   b. 40% to 50%.
   c. 50% to 60%.
   d. 60% to 70%.

174. Ms. Anders must have dialysis or transplantation in order to survive when kidney function falls below
   a. 30% to 40%.
   b. 20% to 30%.
   c. 15% to 20%.
   d. 10% to 15%.

175. Dialysis will likely begin when Ms. Anders has a GFR (Modification of Diet in Renal Disease [MDRD] equation) of
   a. <15 mL/min/1.73 m2.
   b. <20 mL/min/1.73 m2.
   c. <25 mL/min/1.73 m2.
   d. <30 mL/min/1.73 m2.

Answers and Explanations

Section Description: Jones Case

1. C: The psychiatric disorder that is most common in patients with ESKD is depression, which may occur in 10% to 50% of patients on dialysis. One of the primary problems associated with depression is nonadherence because patients who are depressed may feel that compliance with treatment is pointless, or they may be suicidal and feel that they want to die. In fact, suicide rates are higher for dialysis patients than for the general population. Psychiatric problems affect about 10% of hospitalized patients with ESKD.

2. C: If a patient with ESKD is screened with the Beck Depression Inventory (BDI) and has a score of 20, this suggests moderate depression. This tool has 21 items that are scored from 0 (no problem) to 3 (severe). The higher the score, the more severe the depression. BDI is normed for adults between the ages of 17 and 80 years and is often used to screen patients with kidney disease. Scores:
- 0 to 9 no signs of depression
- 10 to 18 mild depression
- 19 to 29 moderate depression
- 30 to 63 severe depression

3. A: For a patient with ESKD, the dosage of an SSRI should be reduced by two-thirds. SSRIs pose an increased risk of bleeding and nausea and vomiting, symptoms that may occur with ESKD, so the patient must be monitored carefully. However, the SSRI may provide some additional benefit by decreasing incidence of postural and intradialytic hypotension because of improved vascular tone. The most common drug prescribed for ESKD patients is fluoxetine (usually 20 mg daily).

4. C: The purpose of a high-carbohydrate diet for a patient with kidney failure is to spare protein for growth and healing. Protein intake must be individualized so that the body's requirements for protein are met while preventing symptoms related to uremia. With a high-carbohydrate diet, the carbohydrates are burned to provide energy for the body while the protein is "spared." Patients may need to limit some high-carbohydrate foods that are also high in potassium, so consultation with a nutritionist is an important part of dietary education.

5. D: The MIA syndrome commonly found in ESKD refers to (1) malnutrition, (2) inflammation, and (3) atherosclerosis. Malnutrition may result from inadequate diet (particularly protein), loss of appetite, GI bleeding, substance abuse, impaired metabolic processes, and factors associated with hemodialysis, such as inadequate Kt/V. Inflammation is related to increased oxidative stress, production of cytokines (interleukin 1β, interleukin 6, tumor necrosis factor), metabolic acidosis, and infection. Atherosclerosis is associated with a variety of factors, including hyperlipidemia and lipoprotein abnormalities.

Section Description: Maddox Case Questions

6. B: When teaching a patient with kidney failure and hemodialysis to manage fluid balance, the nurse advises the patient that a 1 kg (2.2 lb) increase in weight in 24 hours is approximately equivalent to fluid retention of 1 L. Patients should be advised to monitor intake and output and take daily weights. Patients' "dry" weights should be estimated every 3 to 6 weeks in order to help

to estimate weight gain related to fluids. Weight gained between dialysis treatments should not exceed 5% of the dry weight estimate.

7. C: If a patient on hemodialysis has been advised to avoid foods high in phosphorus, dairy products should be limited. Other foods and beverages that are high in phosphorus include beer, ale, colas, chocolate, high-protein meats (liver, organ meats), oysters, sardines, dried beans and peas, nuts, seeds, whole grains, wheat germ, and bran. Normal phosphorus level is 2.5 to 4.5 mg/dL. Lowering phosphorus levels helps to increase absorption of calcium.

8. D: If a patient on hemodialysis has been prescribed sevelamer hydrochloride as a phosphate binder, she should be advised to take this medication with meals. Because sevelamer hydrochloride may bind to other medications and decrease their bioavailability, other drugs should be given an hour before sevelamer or 3 hours after. The dosage of sevelamer should be adjusted to maintain a phosphorus level of 3.5 to 5.5 mg/dL. Calcium, bicarbonate, and chloride levels should be monitored as well as phosphorus.

Section Description: Logan Case Questions

9. A: Chronic kidney disease is staged according to the patient's glomerular filtration rate (GFR). The GFR shows the quantity of glomerular filtrate produced each minute in the nephrons, based on clearance of specific substances. Different equations are used to estimate the GFR, but the National Kidney Foundation Kidney Disease Outcomes Quality Initiative (NKF KDOQI) guidelines recommend the MDRD Study Equation, which is based on the serum creatinine and is normalized to a body surface area of 1.73 m². Thus, the equation does not require the patient's height and weight. The equation requires age and includes adjustments for females and for African Americans.

10. D: As chronic kidney disease progresses from stage 2 to stage 3, the focus of clinical intervention moves toward evaluating and treating complications. The plans for the 5 stages of chronic kidney disease are as follows:
   1. Diagnosing and establishing treatment plan as well as reducing risk of cardiovascular disease and slowing disease progression.
   2. Monitoring the progression of the disease.
   3. Evaluating and treating complications, as kidney function is increasingly impaired.
   4. Preparing the patient for eventual dialysis and/or kidney transplant so that patient understands requirements and options.
   5. Educating and assisting patient to undergo dialysis and, if appropriate, prepare for transplantation.

Section description: Carroll Case Questions

11. C: When using continuous venovenous hemodialysis (CVVHD) for a patient with severe uremia requiring large-volume removal of fluid, the desirable mean arterial pressure (MAP) for optimal fluid removal and dialysis is 70 mm Hg (although many patients who are critically ill may have a lower MAP). For a patient with a BP of 190/100 mm Hg, the formula for MAP is:
- (systolic blood pressure plus 2X the diastolic blood pressure) divided by 3
- MAP = 190 + 200 = 390/3 = 130.

12. C: If a patient is undergoing continuous renal replacement therapy (CRRT) and filter clotting occurs, causing the ultrafiltration rate to slow even after lowering the effluent container, the nurse should assess the system for obstruction or inadequate heparinization. If adjusting the

anticoagulation does not improve the rate of ultrafiltration, the physician should be notified, and the system may need to be replaced. During replacement, the catheters and the new system should be primed with anticoagulated solution.

13. B: If a patient is undergoing continuous venovenous hemodialysis (CVVHD) with heparin used for anticoagulation and the nurse notes blood oozing from the catheter insertion site, the activated clotting time (ACT) should be monitored at least every hour and heparin dose adjusted within established protocol. The dressings should be assessed for blood loss with strict aseptic technique used for vascular access. The patient's vital signs should be monitored carefully and effluent checked for signs of blood.

14. A: If a patient undergoing CRRT becomes hypotensive but the lines are not disconnected and there is no blood leak, the nurse should suspect the cause is an increased ultrafiltration rate. The ultrafiltration rate is the rate at which fluid is removed, and if this occurs too rapidly, the patient may experience a drop in blood pressure. The ultrafiltration rate for CVVHD is 500 to 800 mL/h. With hypotension, the ultrafiltration rate may need to be decreased and/or replacement fluids increased.

15. D: According to the Centers for Disease Control and Prevention (CDC), to reduce the incidence of infection, CRRT catheters should be changed only when clinically indicated. Routine changes of catheters are no longer advised because each change increases the risk of infection. For venovenous access, an uncuffed double lumen catheter is inserted into a large vein, usually the femoral or jugular. The subclavian vein may also be used if the femoral or jugular veins are contraindicated for some reason.

16. C: According to KDIGO AKI guidelines, CRRT is recommended over intermittent hemodialysis specifically for patients with kidney failure and cerebral edema or signs of increased intracerebral pressure. The dialysis or replacement fluid used is more sodium hypertonic (>140 mM) than usual to prevent movement of fluid into the brain. In some cases when the intracranial pressure is uncontrolled, the patient may benefit from cooling of the replacement fluids.

Section Description: Mayer Case Questions

17. B: If a patient with symptoms of acute glomerulonephritis also presents with malar rash, arthralgias, and oral lesions, these findings are suggestive of systemic lupus erythematosus (SLE), which is a common noninfectious cause of acute glomerulonephritis. SLE is a multisystem autoimmune disorder. With SLE, the injury to the glomeruli is related to deposition of immune complexes. Lupus nephritis commonly occurs within 5 years of diagnosis of SLE as the disease progresses. The patient is also at increased risk of cardiovascular disease.

18. D: Based on these findings, the patient may require consultation with a rheumatologist because the treatment approach is different from that used for infectious causes of acute glomerulonephritis. For example, steroids may be indicated for SLE and are contraindicated for infectious glomerulonephritis. Symptoms associated with SLE may be varied, and treatment challenging, so a physician with expertise in treating SLE should be consulted prior to beginning treatment if possible.

Section Description: Independent Questions, Group 1

19. A: Healthcare personnel caring for patients undergoing kidney transplantation should receive an annual influenza immunization. The CDC recommendations for healthcare personnel also include the hepatitis B series, varicella, and measles, mumps, and rubella (MMR) if not already immune, and a single dose of Tdap. Once an adult has received the Tdap vaccination, subsequent boosters should be with Td every 10 years. Family members and caregivers should also be advised to have the same immunizations in order to protect the patient.

20. C: The most common infection following kidney transplantation is urinary tract infections, which include 45% to 47% of infections and impair the function of the donor kidney or lead to loss of the kidney and, in some cases, death. Infection is especially dangerous if it occurs in the first 6 months after transplant. Bacteriuria and UTI may be asymptomatic because of immunosuppression. Administration of antibiotic prophylaxis and early removal of urethral catheters have helped to reduce infections, but rates remain high.

21. D: If, 12 months after receiving a kidney transplant, a patient experiences reduced urinary output and increasing serum creatinine levels and ultrasonography shows hydronephrosis is present, the most likely cause is ureteral stenosis, which has caused urine to back up into the kidney. Ureteral stenosis usually occurs relatively late, months or even years after kidney transplant. Causes may vary, including fibrotic changes, an anastomosis that is too tight, or external compression, such as from a lymphocele.

22. D: If a patient with a donor kidney develops sudden onset of hypertension 2 years after transplantation, the most likely cause is arterial stenosis, which can occur in up to 10% of patients within a few months or years after transplantation. Angiography is usually done to exclude other diagnoses and confirm stenosis. Treatment most commonly involves angioplasty and stent placement in order to ensure patency of the artery. Doppler ultrasonography may be used postoperatively to monitor progress and assess for hematoma formation.

23. A: If, following kidney transplantation, a patient develops a large lymphocele between the bladder and the transplanted kidney, the treatment of choice is usually internal drainage into the abdomen, done laparoscopically. A lymphocele usually develops within the first year when lymphatic vessels leak lymph into the tissues. Patients typically complain of edema and pain and exhibit impairment of renal function. If the lymphocele is very small, sclerotherapy may be used, but the lymphocele may recur. Aspiration may increase risk of infection, especially if a drainage catheter is left in place. Fibrin glue is sometimes used.

24. B: Kidney rejection occurring within hours of transplantation is classified as hyperacute. Types of rejection include:
- Hyperacute: This can occur within a few minutes or hours of transplantation and results from anti-donor antibodies and complement system activation.
- Accelerated: This may occur within days of transplantation and involves reactivation of sensitized T cells.
- Acute: This may occur within days up to a number of weeks and involves primary activation of T cells.
- Chronic: This form develops over a period of months to years and involves multiple factors, both immunologic and nonimmunologic.

25. C: When OKT3 treatment is used for a severe acute kidney rejection episode, premedication usually begins with IV methylprednisolone (250 to 500 mg), which is administered about an hour before administration of OKT3 and again 30 minutes after. Diphenhydramine (50 mg IV) is also usually administered before the OKT3 each day, and acetaminophen (650 mg) is given 30 minutes before. Cyclosporine is discontinued, but azathioprine may be continued (25 mg/day). OKT3 is generally administered at 5 mg/day for 2 weeks.

26. C: According to the RIFLE (Risk, Injury, Failure, Loss of kidney function, ESKD) criteria for acute kidney dysfunction, urinary output indicative of kidney failure is <0.3 mL/kg/h for 24 hours. Other indications include serum creatinine 3 times normal or serum creatinine of ≥4 mg/dL with acute rise in serum creatinine of ≥0.5 mg/dL. The RIFLE criteria are used to determine the risk of developing acute kidney injury (AKI) in patients who are critically ill. The first 3 categories (RIF) indicate increasing severity of disease and the last 2 (LE) indicate outcome criteria.

27. D: Tumor lysis syndrome is an example of an intrarenal cause of acute kidney injury (AKI). AKI may be prerenal, intrarenal, or postrenal, depending on the cause:
- Prerenal: extended hypotension (sepsis, vasodilation), low cardiac output (heart failure, cardiogenic shock), volume depletion (hemorrhage, dehydration), and renovascular thrombosis
- Intrarenal: kidney ischemia, endogenous toxins (rhabdomyolysis, tumor lysis syndrome), exogenous toxins (contrast dyes, nephrotoxic drugs)
- Postrenal: obstruction (ureters, bladder, urethra)

28. B: Many commonly used medications are nephrotoxic, especially if taken in large amounts. Drugs that may cause tubular cell toxicity include aminoglycosides, antiretrovirals, contrast dye, zoledronate, and amphotericin B. Because the proximal tubular cells actively concentrate and reabsorb glomerular filtrate, the cells are exposed to toxic elements. Other pathogenic mechanisms include alterations in intraglomerular hemodynamics, inflammation, crystal nephropathy, rhabdomyolysis, and thrombotic microangiopathy.

29. C: If 200 patients are exposed to an airborne virus carried by a staff member over a 1-week period and 40 patients are infected, the attack rate is 20%. The attack rate shows the proportion of at-risk patients who are exposed and become infected. Attack rates are always calculated as a percentage based on the number of cases per 100. Since there are 20 patients per 100, the calculation is 20/100 X 100 = 20%.

30. B: If an infection involves a propagating source, the nurse would expect the infection to spread from person to person, either through airborne means or through direct contact. With a propagating source, there may be waves of infections because the first infected group infects a subsequent group, so the infection keeps spreading. With a common source, there is one source of infection, such as a water supply, that can directly infect multiple persons. A common source of infection is easier to contain than a propagating source.

31. D: If 4 patients in a community of 2000 people are infected with MRSA, this would be classified as a cluster because of the small number. If the number grows beyond what is expected for the population, it would be classified as an outbreak or epidemic, with the terms often used interchangeably. The term epidemic sometimes refers to a larger spread of the disease. A pandemic occurs when the epidemic spreads very widely, sometimes to multiple countries.

32. A: The risk of disease occurring in a population (such as the number of people with kidney failure who develop a urinary tract infection) over a specified period of time (such as 1 year) is the incidence rate. For example, if there are 500 patients with kidney failure and 42 develop urinary tract infections over the course of 1 year, the numerator is the number of infections and the denominator the total number of patients:
- 42/500 = 0.084 X 100 = 8.4% incidence rate.

Section Description: Aiken Case Questions

33. D: When assisting a surgeon with stencil-based preoperative mapping for insertion of a peritoneal dialysis catheter, the patient should initially be positioned supine so that the abdomen can be easily visualized and the stencil placed in various positions that are appropriate for different catheters and the exit sites marked with a marking pen. Then, the patient is assisted to sitting and standing positions so that the surgeon can evaluate the exit sites in relation to skin folds, creases, and the belt line. When an exit site is selected, then the mapping is completed.

34. D: Prior to surgical placement of a catheter for peritoneal dialysis, the recommended antibiotic prophylaxis is generally a first-generation cephalosporin. Vancomycin is also frequently used, but the issue of antibiotic resistance should be considered carefully and balanced against benefits of vancomycin. Usually, 1 dose of antibiotic is given at the time of the catheter insertion. A double-cuff catheter is recommended because of lower rates of infection and other site complications.

35. C: If a culture of the catheter exit site is positive for *Staphylococcus aureus* but there is no erythema or purulent discharge, the most likely cause of the positive culture is colonization, which frequently occurs within a short time after insertion of the catheter. Colonization is a form of contamination that can lead to more serious infections because colonized bacteria are more resistant to antibiotics. Erythema, by itself, is not always indicative of an infection, while purulent discharge is.

36. A: While not used in a hospital environment, a heating pad may be used to warm dialysate solution in the home environment. Maintaining a stable temperature can be difficult, and warming may take a prolonged period of time. The heating pad should have an automatic shut-off time to prevent overheating (usually about 2 hours). With this method of heating, it is especially important to check the temperature of the solution prior to instillation. Other methods used include warming cabinets and microwave ovens (not recommended but frequently used).

37. B: Once a dialysate bag is heated, the temperature can be assessed by folding the bag over and enclosing an electronic thermometer. The temperature of the dialysate should be at body temperature (37 °C) because instilling room temperature dialysate may result in chills and lowering of the body temperature. The bag should be rotated to mix the solution thoroughly before measuring temperature in case hot spots are present, especially if the dialysate was heated in a microwave oven.

38. C: With continuous ambulatory peritoneal dialysis (CAPD), the number of exchanges in 24 hours is usually 4 to 5 with 3 to 4 done during the daytime hours (every 4 to 6 hours) and one longer exchange done during the night. During the daytime, drainage usually takes about 20 minutes. The dwell time during the night is extended to 8 to 10 hours to allow the patient to sleep. The dextrose concentration of the overnight dwell may be higher than that used during the day because of the longer duration.

39. D: In order to prevent gram-negative catheter-related infections, patients undergoing CAPD should avoid swimming in a lake, river, stream, or public pool, or soaking in a tub because of the bacteria present in the water. Once the exit site is well healed, wearing a dressing is not generally necessary unless the patient is working outside in dusty conditions or doing dirty work, such as farm work, during which covering the exit site with a gauze dressing is a reasonable precaution.

40. C: With CAPD, the volume of dialysate retained in the peritoneal cavity (dwell) at all times in adults is usually approximately ≤2 L. Exchanges are usually carried out every 3 to 4 hours during the day. The dialysate is instilled in about 10 minutes, during which the patient may sit, stand, or lie down. After instillation, the catheter is clamped until the prescribed dwell time is completed and then drained.

Section Description: Elmers Case Questions

41. A: If a patient on hemodialysis is pregnant and her blood pressure is 160/100 mm Hg when euvolemic, an acceptable medication to treat hypertension is labetalol. Atenolol is contraindicated because it is classified as pregnancy risk category D. Both ACE inhibitors and ARBs are associated with congenital abnormalities, including dysplastic kidneys, neonatal anuria, pulmonary hypoplasia, and skull ossification defects. Hydralazine can be given in addition to other medications but should not be used as a single agent.

42. D: In order to increase the chance that the patient on hemodialysis will deliver a viable infant, ideally the pregnant patient should be dialyzed more than 20 hours per week. Intensive dialysis has been shown to decrease premature delivery and increase live births; however, the optimal number of hours per week have not been established. One study showed that most infants survived when the mother had 48 hours of dialysis per week. Both increased PD and hemodialysis increase survival rates, but it is more difficult to increase the hours of PD.

Section Description: Stephens Case Questions

43. A: In a patient with chronic kidney failure and impaired cognition because of increased BUN and creatinine levels, the priority for patient education should be dietary and fluid restrictions in order to help control BUN and creatinine levels. These needs take priority because they are related to the patient's physiological condition. Hygiene and exercise needs may also be addressed. Because the patient has mildly impaired cognition, detailed information about the pathophysiology of the disease may be more difficult to comprehend.

44. A: With chronic renal failure, specific gravity usually ranges from 1.007 to 1.01 with urine isotonic to plasma at all times (regardless of fluid intake or time of day) because the nephrons have hypertrophied in an effort to compensate for the kidney damage, and they are unable to adequately filter waste products. With normal kidney function, specific gravity is usually about 1.015 but may vary widely from 1.001 to 1.04 depending on intake of fluid and other substances, such as sodium and protein.

45. A: If a patient's cardiac output decreases, resulting in arterial hypoperfusion with reduced blood flow to the kidneys, the nurse expects lab results to show increased BUN because the reduced blood flow reduces glomerular filtration and urinary output, allowing the BUN to increase. If perfusion is restored quickly, then the kidneys may not have permanent damage; if perfusion is not restored quickly, significant irreversible renal damage may occur. This type of prerenal AKI is common in patients with critical illness.

46. D: In elderly patients with kidney failure, the first signs of various types of infection may be confusion and incontinence. Urinary infections, especially, are associated with sudden onset of confusion in older adults. Dehydration, which is also common in older adults with infection and fever, may also lead to confusion. The overall confusion associated with infection makes older adults more prone to incontinence, especially if the infection involves the urinary tract.

47. A: Prior to a serum creatinine test, the patient should be advised to avoid excessive exercise because creatinine is a product of muscle metabolism, and excessive exercise may cause a sudden increase. About 98% of creatinine is in the muscles, and virtually all of it is excreted through the kidneys. Thus, if the kidney tubules are impaired, the serum creatinine level rises. Creatinine is monitored daily to determine if kidney function is stable, decreasing, or increasing.

48. A: With kidney disease, decreased specific gravity may result from volume excess and intrarenal acute kidney injury. Decreased specific gravity occurs when the kidneys are not able to adequately excrete solutes. Increased specific gravity, on the other hand, results from volume deficit, glycosuria, and proteinuria as well as prerenal acute kidney injury. Specific gravity is the measure of the water by weight in comparison to distilled water (which has a specific gravity of 1.000), so the more solutes in the urine, the greater the specific gravity. Normal values range from 1.005 to 1.03.

Section Description: Independent Questions, Group 2

49. C: The primary preventive measure to avoid contrast-induced nephrotoxic injury for a patient who must receive IV radiopaque contrast material despite chronic kidney dysfunction is IV normal saline. Hydration should be carried out aggressively both during the procedure and after. In some cases, patients may be able to hydrate orally by drinking several liters of water over 12 hours. Avoiding dehydration is critical. N-acetylcysteine and fenoldopam have not been shown to provide additional benefit, and studies on the benefit of adding sodium bicarbonate have been inconclusive.

50. D: African Americans are the ethnic group that is most at risk for development of kidney failure, accounting for about a third of the cases in the United States. African Americans have high rates of both hypertension and diabetes mellitus, both of which increase the risk of kidney damage. Other groups that have increased risk of kidney failure are Hispanic Americans (twice the risk of Caucasians), Asian Americans, Pacific Islanders, and Native Americans. These ethnic groups also have high rates of diabetes and hypertension.

51. B: If the goal is to utilize a simple display of data to show patients and staff progress in decreasing infections in patients with kidney disease each month over the past year, the best display type is likely a line graph. The line graph is uncluttered, easily understood by most people, and requires little or no understanding of statistical measures. It may be presented as a simple one line run chart or as a control chart, which includes a goal and/or median line showing upper and lower parameters.

52. C: The FDA, through the Center for Biologics Evaluation and Research (CBER), is the agency responsible for the safety of the nation's blood supply and sets standards for blood collection, testing, and distribution. CBER also regulates cell separation devices and blood collection containers as well as screening tests, such as for HIV. Additionally, the FDA sets standards for and regulates medical devices and equipment, including dialysis machines.

53. D: If a patient with chronic kidney failure develops pyelonephritis, the antibiotic of choice is generally a fluoroquinolone, such as ciprofloxacin. Ciprofloxacin has good penetration of tissue so the concentration of antibiotic is adequate. Cephalosporins may be used as the second-line drug. Aminoglycosides increase risk of nephrotoxicity and are generally avoided. Patients with chronic kidney failure are at increased risk of adverse effects from penicillins.

54. A: The primary complication from recurrent pyelonephritis is scarring, which can lead to reduced kidney function and chronic kidney failure. Recurrent pyelonephritis is more common in children than adults and is often associated with vesicoureteral reflux (VUR), which may be undetected before damage occurs. Females are more likely to contract pyelonephritis than males, and pregnancy may cause the kidney damage to progress. Hypertension also has a negative effect on the kidneys, causing further deterioration of function.

55. C: Following a percutaneous kidney biopsy, the most common complication is hematuria. While bleeding is usually not severe and clears within a few days, in some cases hemorrhage may occur, so patients should be advised to monitor urinary output and report excessive bleeding or bright red blood. Pain is usually mild. If the biopsy needle is inadvertently inserted into an adjacent artery and vein, an AV fistula may form, but it usually closes without intervention. Hematomas rarely occur but may become infected.

56. B: In response to decreased renal blood flow and decreased pressure in the glomerulus, renin is released and enters general circulation where it is converted to angiotensin I and then angiotensin II, which causes vasoconstriction and increased vascular resistance, which in turn decreases renin again. Angiotensin II also causes aldosterone release, which increases sodium and fluid reabsorption. This increases renal blood flow and blood volume, which increase pressure in the glomerulus. This then also decreases renin.

57. A: Nephrotic syndrome is characterized by marked proteinuria (greater than 3.5 g/day) because of increased glomerulus permeability. The proteinuria is mirrored by resultant hypoalbuminemia, and the albumin is filtered out of the blood and excreted. Other characteristics include diffuse pitting edema (about the eyes and in dependent areas) and hyperlipidemia. Treatment usually includes diuretics, ACE inhibitors, and lipid-lowering agents.

58. C: Patients may be advised to fast for at least 4 hours prior to a CT of the kidney with IV iodinated contrast because they may experience nausea and vomiting. These adverse effects usually last only for a few moments, but patients who have recently eaten food are more likely to vomit. Patients with chronic kidney disease are especially at risk for contrast-induced nephropathy and should have volume expansion before and after the CT either through oral or IV fluids.

59. A: The primary causes of nephrosclerosis are hypertension and diabetes. Nephrosclerosis results in hardening of the renal arteries and is a main cause of chronic kidney disease and ESKD. In younger adults, malignant nephrosclerosis occurs with significant hypertension and is more common in males than females. The impaired perfusion of the kidney results in necrotic areas and fibrosis, leading to uremia. Benign nephrosclerosis occurs in older adults who have hypertension and atherosclerosis.

60. C: If, shortly after admission for post-infectious acute glomerulonephritis, the patient develops altered mental status, the most likely cause of this complication is hypertensive encephalopathy. This may occur with acute glomerulonephritis and is an emergent condition that requires immediate treatment with vasodilators/antihypertensives. Infections that may precipitate acute

glomerulonephritis include group A beta-hemolytic streptococcal infection (usually pharyngitis) and numerous viral infections, including Epstein-Barr, hepatitis B, and HIV.

61. D: Prerenal kidney failure, which is associated with renal hypoperfusion, may result from volume depletion, which may be caused by severe dehydration, hemorrhage, diuresis (sometimes related to diuretics), vomiting, diarrhea, and NG suctioning. Other causes of prerenal failure include impaired cardiovascular functioning, such as may occur with MI, heart failure, cardiac dysrhythmias, and cardiogenic shock. Prerenal kidney failure may also result from marked vasodilation that occurs with sepsis, anaphylaxis, and antihypertensive medications.

62. A: Characteristic of acute prerenal kidney failure is sodium level of less than 20 mEq/L compared with more than 40 mEq/L for intrarenal renal failure. BUN and serum creatinine are increased, similar to intrarenal kidney failure, while urinary output is decreased with prerenal and increased with intrarenal. Urine sediment is usually within normal parameters with a few hyaline casts with prerenal failure while abnormal casts and debris are common with intrarenal. Urine osmolality is more than 500 mOsm/L with prerenal failure and less than 350 mOsm/L with intrarenal. Specific gravity is increased with prerenal and low normal with intrarenal.

63. B: The obligatory urine output (minimal amount of urinary output) that is needed to filter normal metabolic waste products and remove them from the body is about 500 mL. Normal kidneys must be able to excrete urine ranging from very dilute to very concentrated, as this is necessary to regulate serum sodium and fluid balance. Kidneys normally excrete a solute load of 600 to 800 mOsm/day. The maximum capacity of the kidneys to concentrate urine is 1200 mOsm/L, so if a patient has solute excretion of 600 mOsm (half his maximum capacity), the minimal urine output is 0.5 L (500 mL).

64. D: The medication that is nephrotoxic and should have baseline and follow-up BUN and serum creatinine monitored during administration is vancomycin. Numerous medications may be nephrotoxic, but medications with increased risk that require monitoring include aminoglycosides, gentamicin, tobramycin, cyclosporine, amphotericin B, and polymyxin B. ACE inhibitors should be discontinued or carefully monitored if serum creatinine levels are significantly elevated. Some diuretics commonly used in treatment of kidney failure, such as furosemide, may also have nephrotoxic properties.

65. B: If a patient with kidney failure has an order for a sodium polystyrene sulfonate (Kayexalate) retention enema, the nurse expects that the patient is being treated for hyperkalemia (value greater than 5.5 mEq/L). Hyperkalemia is characterized by diarrhea, generalized muscle weakness, abdominal cramping, slurred speech, dyspnea, and paresthesia. ECG abnormalities, such as peaked T waves, may occur, increasing the risk of cardiac arrest if hyperkalemia is not promptly treated and reversed.

66. D: If a patient with acute renal failure is stabilizing and seems alert and responsive, but the nurse notes that the patient needs to have explanations for treatment and procedures repeated many times, the most likely reason is anxiety. Acute kidney failure may cause severe anxiety because of the intensive treatment, including dialysis, which may be needed to stabilize the patient; the patient may be inundated with information and decisions. Patients may have difficulty concentrating and remembering details.

67. B: According to KDIGO AKI guidelines, CRRT for patients with AKI should deliver effluent volume of 20 to 25 mL/h, although some studies seem to suggest that higher volumes render better

outcomes. The inflow rate may need to be decreased to reach this target because up to 5 L/day of excess fluid may be removed from the patient, but lowering the inflow rate too much may lead to partial clotting of the dialyzer.

68. D: If a new nurse in the critical care unit is unfamiliar with CRRT equipment being used and works very slowly because of the need to check procedures, the best solution is to offer to assist and mentor the new nurse. Working one-on-one with an experienced nurse is often the best way to improve skills and can also decrease risks to the patients because being unfamiliar with equipment can lead to errors.

69. D: Slow continuous ultrafiltration (SCUF), a form of continuous renal replacement therapies, removes fluids at the rate of 100 to 300 mL/h but does not replace fluids. SCUF can be used for patients with generalized edema associated with heart failure or those with decreased renal perfusion nonresponsive to diuretics, but SCUF is not commonly used. If a patient experiences fluid deficit, then intravenous fluids must be administered to compensate for excess fluid loss.

Section Description: Mayweather Case Questions

70. C: If a patient who has been treated for kidney failure with hemodialysis for 5 years has developed pain and stiffness in the joints, the most likely cause is amyloidosis. This typically occurs after about 5 years of treatment because hemodialysis is not able to adequately filter amyloid proteins out of the blood as effectively as healthy kidneys. Amyloid proteins build up in organs and in joints and tendons, and the deposits damage the joints. Treatment is palliative only; there is no effective treatment or cure.

71. D: If a patient with kidney failure complains of severe itching during and after hemodialysis despite taking a phosphate binder, diphenhydramine (Benadryl) is commonly prescribed and may relieve itching for some patients. Some patients also find relief from hydroxyzine (Atarax). Ultraviolet light exposure through direct sunlight or light box may also reduce itching. If itching is unremitting, some patients have part of their parathyroid glands removed to reduce the increased levels of parathyroid hormone, which may cause itching.

72. A: A primary advantage of home hemodialysis is the ability to do more frequent treatments. At hemodialysis centers, treatments are usually done for 3 to 4 hours three times a week; with home hemodialysis, the patient can take shorter daily treatments so there is less fluid and waste buildup in the body, lowering the risk of complications. Patients are able to schedule treatments at their own convenience, giving them more freedom to live their lives. While costs remain high, patients may save expenses related to travel, especially if the center is far away.

73. D: The most important factor for creation of a buttonhole tracks for hemodialysis is that the same cannulator does all treatments until the tunnel is established, and this can take up to 10 cannulations in patients who are good healers or 14 for patients who are slow healers, such as diabetic patients. The original cannulator should carefully document the insertion site and the angle of insertion and should ideally supervise subsequent cannulators. When possible, patients should be taught to self-cannulate once the tunnel is well established.

74. B: If using a combination chlorhexidine gluconate and alcohol skin prep (such as ChloraPrep) before cannulation, the skin contact time required is 30 seconds. Then the prep should be allowed to dry thoroughly (up to 3 minutes on hairless skin) before cannulation. Alcohol prep used alone

also should have skin contact of 30 seconds. Povidone iodine prep (such as Betadine), however, requires a longer contact time of at least 3 minutes.

75. C: If a patient on home hemodialysis has buttonhole tracks, after the area is cleansed and prepped for treatment, the next step is to use a scab picker/aseptic tweezers to remove the scabs that form over the opening of the tracts. Once these are removed, dull needles are inserted into the tracks for the treatment. Using the treatment needle to remove scabs increases risk of infection. Buttonhole tracks form literal tunnels to the vein. The tunnels stay open, much like a pierced ear.

76. B: Following home dialysis for a patient with buttonhole tracks, the patient should be taught to apply firm pressure with 2 fingers as the needles are removed and then to maintain the pressure for 5 to 10 minutes after, depending on how long it takes for a clot to form. Because the buttonhole track is open, if the patient removes the needle without applying pressure with a gauze pad, blood will spurt freely out of the track.

77. C: If a patient with buttonhole access for hemodialysis frequently has long clots that are very difficult to remove, the most likely reason is failure to use 2-finger hold for needle removal. It is important when removing the needle to apply pressure to both the opening into the skin and the opening into the fistula using 2 fingers, which should easily span both openings. If the opening into the fistula is not compressed, blood will leak into the tunnel, forming a large clot.

78. A: With buttonhole access sites, the cannulator should leave 1/16th to 1/8th inch of the needle exposed to prevent "hubbing." Hubbing occurs when the hub of the needle presses against the buttonhole access site or imbeds into the site, causing the opening to dilate and form a bowl shape, increasing the risk of infection. Because a larger clot may form within the hubbed area, the clot may be difficult to completely remove and the site is more difficult to clean. Additionally, hubbing may result in damage to the epithelial lining of the tunnel.

79. A: The amount of dialysis that a hemodialysis patient is prescribed is based on the removal of urea. Both the removal of urea and the serum level should be monitored, but the removal level is more important than the serum level. Serum levels may at times be within normal ranges even though removal is inadequate (and vice versa) because the rate of urea generation varies from patient to patient depending on many factors, including nutritional status.

80. D: The most common predisposing factor for muscle cramping during hemodialysis is hypotension. Other factors may include hypovolemia, high ultrafiltration rate because of excessive weight gain, and low sodium dialysate. All of these factors may result in vasoconstriction and decreased perfusion to the muscles and cramping. Cramping is more likely to occur in the first weeks of dialysis. In some cases, cramping may be related to hypocalcemia.

81. D: Indications of clotting in the extracorporeal circuit include blood foaming followed by clot formation in the drip chamber and the venous trap. Other indications include blood that is very dark in color; shadows or black streaks in the dialyzer; teetering in the venous line segment past the dialyzer, preventing the blood from entering the venous chamber and causing it to flow back into the line segment; and clots in the inflow dialyzer header. Analyzing pressure readings may help to locate clots that are occlusive.

82. C: Foam in the venous of blood line of a dialyzer may indicate air embolism. While an air embolism may be venous or arterial, venous is more common and may result from system leaks, insertion of central venous catheter, or air in dialysate. If the patient is seated, the air embolism

may enter the cerebral circulation, causing severe neurological impairment. If the patient is lying down, the air embolism may enter the heart and lungs, resulting in cardiac arrhythmias and respiratory distress.

Section Description: Bell Case Questions

83. D: If the partner of a patient with ESKD has volunteered as a living donor, the first concern when evaluating the donor is the person's psychological status because if he or she does not pass this assessment, further assessment is unnecessary. When a family member or partner is involved, then it is very important to ascertain if there is a history of domestic abuse or circumstances that suggest coercion. The potential donor should be assessed for a history of psychiatric or psychological disorders as well as a history of substance abuse.

84. B: Pre-transplant screening for varicella-zoster virus antibody is recommended for adult recipients of a donor kidney. All recipients should also be screened for a history of or exposure to tuberculosis. Patients should have their immunization history reviewed and should receive recommended immunizations prior to transplantation if they are not up to date in order to prevent post-transplant infection. Recommended immunizations include influenza, hepatitis A and B, tetanus, polio, pneumonia, and meningitis.

85. C: Increased morbidity and mortality post-kidney transplant are associated with BMI of greater than 30 kg/m². These increases may result from other factors associated with excess weight, including high rates of diabetes mellitus, hypertension, dyslipidemia, and coronary heart disease. Additionally, patients with higher BMIs are often more sedentary. Patients who are obese should be advised to eat a healthy diet and exercise to tolerance to try to reduce BMI to a healthier level before transplantation.

86. B: The information gleaned during a psychiatric consultation that is most likely to be a contraindication for kidney transplant is a history of nonadherence to treatment regimen. If the patient was unable to adhere to treatment during kidney failure, the patient is likely to encounter problems after transplantation when following the treatment regimen is critical. Patients must demonstrate adherence for a minimal period of 6 months before reconsideration. Many patients have a history of psychiatric disorders, but this alone is not a contraindication, nor is a history of substance abuse or unemployment.

87. B: Following kidney transplantation, fluids must be administered for both maintenance and replacement. Insensible loss is approximately 30 mL/h and is usually replaced with dextrose 5% in water, while other fluid losses, such as from urinary output and NG drainage, are commonly replaced with one-half normal saline. IV fluids are used to help control urinary output, so if urinary output is low, the patient may be administered a bolus of 500 mL to 1 liter of normal saline. Electrolytes are generally provided, if needed, in a separate infusion.

88. D: In the immediate postoperative period after kidney transplantation, the physician should be notified if urinary output is less than 60 mL/h for 2 consecutive hours, more than 300 mL/h for 4 hours, or more than 500 mL/h for 2 consecutive hours. Urinary output must be carefully monitored to assess kidney function and to determine the amount of replacement IV fluids required.

89. B: If, following kidney transplantation, a patient develops a small bladder leak, initial treatment usually includes insertion of a Foley catheter into the bladder and decompression to allow the lesion time to heal spontaneously. Large leaks or those that are located more proximal to the

transplanted kidney may require surgical repair. Leaks may occur throughout the urinary tract after transplantation. The patient may complain of abdominal pain or exhibit edema of the perineal area as well as urinary leakage. The Foley catheter may be gently irrigated with 30 mL normal saline if necessary when clots are present and may be obstructing the lumen.

90. A: Cyclosporine, an immunosuppressive agent used to prevent kidney rejection after transplantation, can be especially nephrotoxic, so kidney function must be monitored carefully during administration. Nephrotoxicity increases with a number of drug-drug interactions (such as with NSAIDs, ranitidine, and many antibiotics), so patients should be advised to always consult with the physician before taking any medications, including OTC. Patients should also avoid St. John's wort, alfalfa sprouts, and grapefruit.

91. A: When a patient is discharged after kidney transplantation, the nurse should ensure the patient understands that the primary measures to determine the health of the kidney are serum creatinine and urinary output. Patients should keep a log of urinary output and should be aware of their serum creatinine levels, so that if patients see local physicians who are less familiar with kidney transplants, the patients can alert the physicians to levels of concern. Any increase of 25% or more in the serum creatinine requires immediate assessment of kidney function.

92. C: The most common complication associated with core needle biopsy of a transplanted kidney is bleeding and hematuria, although the hematuria is usually transient and causes no long-term complications. However, sometimes bleeding may persist, requiring transfusions. Frank hemorrhage is rare. With bleeding, a Foley catheter may be inserted into the bladder to help drain clots. Core biopsies are done to diagnose the cause of graft dysfunction and also for routine monitoring for subclinical graft rejection.

93. A: If a patient exhibits signs of depression post-kidney transplantation, the medicine of choice is usually an SSRI. SSRIs are usually fairly well tolerated by kidney transplant patients and have fewer adverse effects compared with other choices, such as MAO inhibitors or TCAs. St. John's wort interacts with cyclosporine, an immunosuppressive drug usually administered after transplantation. Patients must be monitored very carefully. Some studies show that sertraline may affect cyclosporine concentration, but other SSRIs (such as citalopram, paroxetine, and fluoxetine) do not appear to affect cyclosporine.

Section Description: Independent Questions, Group 3

94. C: The greatest risk of bacteremia occurs with dialysis catheters with the overall infection risk 7 times greater than for patients with an arteriovenous fistula. If a patient is not a candidate for an AV fistula, then an AV graft should be the next choice. Dialysis catheters should be used only for acute dialysis with an expected duration of fewer than 3 weeks; if a longer time is required, then the catheter should be tunneled and cuffed with insertion in the right internal jugular vein.

95. C: Chlorhexidine gluconate 2% is the antiseptic with the broadest spectrum antibacterial activity used for skin prep for a fistula site, and this solution is recommended by the CDC. The solution should be applied back and forth (not in a circle) on the site for 30 seconds as this is the time needed for activation. Antisepsis persists for up to 48 hours after cleansing. The solution should air dry. In some cases, chlorhexidine gluconate 2% is combined with isopropyl alcohol 70%. If used alone, alcohol must be applied for 1 minute and povidone iodine for 2 to 3 minutes.

96. A: If a patient develops an infection of a primary AV fistula and requires more than 6 weeks of antibiotic treatment, subacute endocarditis should be expected. Risk increases with the presence of a calcified valve, a common finding after about 5 years of dialysis treatments. Some patients may be treated solely with antibiotics, but others may require valve replacement because the valve has become so damaged. Commonly found causative agents include *Staphylococcus aureus* and MRSA.

97. C: While a patient is undergoing hemodialysis, chloramine testing should be conducted every 4 hours. Carbon filters are used to remove chloramine, chorine, and organic material from public water supplies. If the chloramine is not removed, it can result in red blood cell hemolysis. The carbon filters may become contaminated with bacteria. Water should be warmed and at least 2 carbon filters used in a series. Prior to testing, the system should be functioning for at least 15 minutes with testing done after the first carbon tank.

98. A: The last component of the water processing system before the distribution loop should be an ultrafilter, which is used with or without ultraviolet lights to remove bacteria and endotoxins from the water supply used for dialysis. In some cases, an ultrafilter may also be placed before the reverse osmosis. Even with the ultrafilters in place, the water supply must be monitored for bacteria and endotoxins because ultrafilters do not remove 100% of all contaminants.

99. B: Fluoride contamination of water used for hemodialysis may result in ventricular fibrillation, which can lead to cardiac arrest. Other symptoms of excessive fluoride include bone disease, pruritus, nausea and vomiting, and chest pain. Fluoride contamination results from inadequate treatment of water. The acceptable level of fluoride is 0.2 ppm, but the level can increase, for example, if a deionizer is exhausted. A deionizer should have both audio and visual alarms, and all staff should be trained to understand the monitoring system in use.

100. B: After implantation of a prosthetic arteriovenous graft, maturation usually takes 3 to 6 weeks; some graft material can be used as soon as the graft has healed, after about 2 weeks. The AV graft is usually done when a patient lacks adequate vessels for formation of an AV fistula. The AV graft is easier to access than an AV fistula but has a shorter life expectancy and is more prone to complications. The graft may be straight or looped.

101. D: Aluminum, which is a contaminant that can be found in water used for dialysis, may result in dialysis dementia. Aluminum toxicity may occur with chronic kidney disease and in patients receiving aluminum-containing dialysate (associated with the aluminum content of the water) and taking aluminum salts as treatment for hyperphosphatemia. Patients may develop encephalopathy, first characterized by difficulties with speech and then dementia, seizures, and myoclonus. Excess aluminum may also cause anemia, osteomalacia, and osteodystrophy.

102. A: If a dialysis patient presents with shaking chills, high fever, myalgia, hypotension, nausea, and vomiting, the most likely causative agents are gram-negative bacteria. Sources of possible contamination include the water processing system, hemodialyzer reprocessing/priming, and ultrafilter waste disposal. Internal sources of gram-negative bacteria, such as perforation of the bowel, should be eliminated. Less commonly, endotoxins may cause a similar reaction with hypotension, fever, and chills, and may progress to multiple organ failure.

103. B: If a patient with acute tubular necrosis is receiving hemodialysis, the phase of the disease that may be obscured is diuresis. Typically, output during this phase is 2 to 4 L, but since excess fluid volume is removed by dialysis, the polyuria is not evident. Phases of acute tubular necrosis include:
- Onset (hours to days): GFR decreases in response to ischemia.
- Oliguric/Anuric (5 to 8 days if nonoliguric and 10 to 16 days if oliguric): GFR decreases and azotemia occurs.
- Diuretic (7 to 14 days): Kidneys clear fluid but not solutes because of scarring and edema of tubules.
- Recovery: GFR slowly recovers.

104. B: If a postmenopausal hemodialysis patient complains of dyspareunia, the most effective treatment is likely sustained-release intravaginal estrogen ring, which has fewer adverse effects than conjugated estrogen cream. The estrogen cream is associated with vaginal bleeding and pain and breast tenderness. Oral estrogen is rarely used with women on hemodialysis. If used, a low dose is needed because the oral estrogen is metabolized more slowly due to the dialysis.

105. D: For a hemodialysis cannulation with a blood flow rate of less than 300 mL/min, the needle gauge size that is usually recommended is 17. The faster the blood flow rate, the larger the needle size (and lower the gauge). For blood flow rates of 300 to 350 mL/min, a 16-gauge needle is recommended. If the blood flow rate increases to 350 to 450 mL/min, a 15-gauge needle is recommended and, for blood flow rates of more than 450 mL/min, a 14-gauge needle.

106. A: The use of topical anesthetics, such as EMLA, to reduce discomfort during cannulation is contraindicated for buttonhole sites because the topical anesthetics should be used only on intact skin. Even when used on intact skin, the topical anesthetic should be used only for 1 to 2 weeks and not for long-term cannulation. EMLA is usually applied to the skin and covered with an airtight dressing or plastic wrap and left in place for at least an hour before needle sticks.

107. A: If a dialysis center is utilizing Continuous Quality Improvement methods, the question that the nurse should continually ask is, "How can the center do things better?" The emphasis with CQI is more on process and improving processes to improve efficiency rather than on individuals. CQI focuses on both the needs of internal customers (such as staff) and external customers (such as patients) and is data-driven. CQI also stresses the point that improvement can occur with small steps and should be the concern of all staff rather than just administration.

108. C: Early symptoms of disequilibrium syndrome associated with long-term hemodialysis include headache, nausea, and vomiting. While the cause is not clear, it may be due to increased cerebral edema. Acutely uremic patients undergoing hemodialysis may exhibit more severe symptoms, including seizures and coma. Mild cases may be treated symptomatically, but if patients are acutely uremic, the blood flow rate may need to be slowed or dialysis discontinued.

109. A: If an 80-year-old patient with ESKD is a candidate for hemodialysis, but the patient refuses treatment, the nurse should respect the patient's decision, recognizing that patients have a legal and moral right to self-determination. The Patient Self-Determination Act specifically gives people the right to refuse treatment and requires that hospitals and other healthcare facilities and organizations provide information about advance directives to ensure patients' wishes are respected.

110. C: If a patient with diabetes mellitus at high risk for kidney disease shows negative results for macroscopic protein with dipstick testing, the nurse expects the next step to be testing for microalbuminuria because early diagnosis is essential to prevent further deterioration of function. Serum creatinine may remain normal until the GRF has fallen to less than 60 mL/min/1.73 m². Normal albumin excretion is 2 to 30 mg/day while microalbuminuria is 30 to 300 mg/day and macroalbuminuria is greater than 300 mg/day.

111. A: When teaching a patient on hemodialysis to manage fluid intake, the nurse advises the patient that fluid intake should be based on 1000 mL/day (this may vary according to individuals) plus the amount of urine in the preceding 24-hour period, in this case 500 mL. Thus, the patient is allowed 1500 mL/day intake. As the time lengthens between treatments, fluid retention usually increases and urinary output decreases, so fluid intake is increasingly restricted.

112. B: If a patient who usually drinks 2 cups of caffeinated coffee daily has headaches during hemodialysis, the patient should be advised to drink a cup of strong coffee with treatment to compensate for the lack of caffeine during hemodialysis. The patient is likely experiencing caffeine withdrawal. As an alternative, the patient can transition to decaffeinated beverages. Taking acetaminophen at the beginning of treatment may help to prevent or control the headaches.

113. D: The agency that sets the minimally adequate target spKt/V (currently 1.4) as a clinical performance measure for all out-patient dialysis centers in the United States is the Centers for Medicare and Medicaid Services (CMS), based on the NKF KDOQI guidelines. CMS was required by the Balanced Budget Act to establish measures to determine the quality of renal dialysis services paid for by Medicare/Medicaid.

114. C: If the electronic event reporting documentation form for the dialysis center is lengthy and time-consuming and not always applicable to the dialysis unit, the best solution is to identify those elements of the form that need modification. Electronic records can usually be modified to some extent to meet the needs of different departments, so the staff should meet with computer technologists who manage the electronic records.

115. A: All hemodialysis patients should be screened for insomnia because up to 50% of patients have some degree of insomnia, which can adversely affect their quality of life and their abilities to interact socially and carry out activities of daily living. Patients are at increased risk of accidents, and many experience increased depression because of the lack of adequate sleep. The causes of insomnia may be physical or psychosocial, or some combination. Dialysis patients are also at increased risk of other sleep disorders, such as restless legs syndrome, obstructive sleep apnea, and periodic limb movements in sleep.

116. A: If a sentinel event, such as a death resulting from exsanguination, occurs, the initial response must include conducting a root cause analysis to determine where the processes failed and whether standards of care were met. Root cause analysis is done retrospectively to determine causes and may involve review of records, interviews, and observations. The focus should be on identifying the process that failed rather than assigning blame. A review of literature should also be included to review current best practices.

117. C: If patient on hemodialysis had an MI and remains weak but has not resumed any exercise because of fear of another MI, the patient may benefit the most from a referral to cardiac rehabilitation program. Cardiac rehabilitation programs often offer support services, such as counseling and peer groups, as well as physical recovery services, such as physical and/or

occupational therapy, tailored to the patient's abilities and needs. Patients may feel more secure in a sheltered environment when beginning an exercise program.

Section Description: Evans Case Questions

118. C: Application of mupirocin cream or ointment to the exit site may be indicated to prevent exit-site infections for patients who are colonized with *Staphylococcus aureus* while undergoing peritoneal dialysis. However, it is important to ensure that mupirocin is compatible with the catheter material before application, and resistance can occur with prolonged use. Exit-site care should be carried out daily, including cleansing the site with an antiseptic, such as chlorhexidine gluconate 1%.

119. B: For a patient undergoing peritoneal dialysis, when sending a sample of cloudy dialysate for culture and sensitivities, the minimal sample size is 10 mL. Ideally, the sample should be processed immediately, but if processing must be delayed, the sample can be stored at 4 °C for up to 6 hours. Only cloudy dialysate should be cultured, and incubation may require up to a week. Dialysate cultures are frequently negative in the presence of peritonitis, likely because of inadequate culture techniques.

120. D: Minimal diagnostic criteria for peritonitis in a patient undergoing peritoneal dialysis usually includes tenderness around the catheter site and purulent discharge, as well as at least 2 of the following: abdominal pain, dialysate WBC count of greater than 100 cells/mm³ and 50 PMN leukocytes, cloudy dialysate, and positive culture or gram stain of the dialysate. Infections associated with peritoneal dialysis include exit-site infection (erythema, purulent and/or sanguinous drainage, tenderness, edema around exit site), subcutaneous tunnel infections (erythema, edema, purulent discharge, or cellulitis), and peritonitis.

121. A: The most common pathogen isolated from patients with peritoneal dialysis-associated peritonitis is coagulase-negative *Staphylococcus.* Other organisms that are frequently found include *Staphylococcus aureus* and streptococci. Exit-site infections are most commonly caused by staphylococci and *Pseudomonas aeruginosa* while tunnel infections are most commonly caused by *Staphylococcus aureus, Pseudomonas aeruginosa,* and Enterobacteriaceae.

122. A: If a patient is being treated for peritonitis and fibrinous clots are visible in the dialysis effluent, the treatment of choice is heparin, administered intraperitoneally. Fibrin formation is often associated with the onset of peritonitis but it may also occur occasionally as part of routine peritoneal dialysis. Small amounts of the heparin may be absorbed systemically but most is not. However, the heparin may cause a local reaction in which damage may occur to mesothelial cells. Heparin may interfere with the action of rifampin but is compatible with most antibiotics.

Section Description: Walker Case Questions

123. B: Nonadherence to treatment plans is quite common in patients with kidney failure, especially younger patients or those with limited social support because of the limitations treatment poses. The best approach is to avoid criticizing or giving advice but to ask the patient how the nurse can help her better manage her condition. This approach shows respect for the patient as an adult who is free to make her own decisions about treatment and engages her in a cooperative process of change.

124. B: Adult polycystic kidney disease (PKD) is an autosomal dominant disorder, so a patient of childbearing age with this disease may be referred to a genetics counselor when considering pregnancy because the disease may be passed on to children. Pregnant patients are also at increased risk of preeclampsia. PKD causes cysts to form in the kidneys, and sometimes other organs, such as the liver. Patients often develop hypertension, chronic pain, mitral valve prolapse, and diverticulosis, and some progress to kidney failure.

125. A: If a nurse feels a special friendship toward a kidney failure patient who reminds the nurse of a close family member, the nurse should deal with this by acknowledging the feeling. It is not unusual to feel more positively or more negatively toward some patients than others, so the important factor is the ability to recognize these biases and to act in a professional manner, providing the same level of attention and care to all patients.

Section Description: Garcia Case Questions

126. B: If a patient is receiving hemodialysis with a 17-gauge needle but has a blood flow rate of 450 mL/min, the needle is too small for the flow rate, and this can result in hemolysis, which is characterized by chest tightness, back pain, and dyspnea, as well as deepening skin color and port-wine appearing blood in the venous line. If a blood sample is centrifuged, the plasma may be pink-tinged because of the breakdown of red blood cells.

127. C: Based on the patient's symptoms, the immediate action should be to stop the blood pump and clamp the blood lines. The hemolyzed blood should be discarded and not reinfused back into the patient. The hemolysis may continue even after dialysis is discontinued, so the patient must be monitored very carefully. The hematocrit may show a marked decrease if hemolysis is extensive. Hemolysis may also occur if there is obstruction or kinking of the arterial blood line.

128. A: The patient should be carefully monitored for hyperkalemia because the hemolysis releases potassium from the red blood cells, and the serum potassium level may increase, putting the patient at risk for muscle weakness and ECG abnormalities that can lead to cardiac arrest. The patient may require additional dialysis or sodium/potassium ion exchange resin orally or rectally to decrease potassium level. Potassium levels:
- Normal values: 3.5 to 5.5 mEq/L
- Hypokalemia: <3.5 mEq/L; Critical value: <2.5 mEq/L
- Hyperkalemia: >5.5 mEq/L; Critical value: >6.5 mEq/L

129. C: According to NKF KDOQI guidelines, patients receiving hemodialysis (or peritoneal dialysis) should receive treatment with an active vitamin D sterol (such as calcitriol) when parathyroid hormone (PTH) levels are greater than 300 pg/mL. Calcitriol is usually administered IV because oral calcitriol is less effective. Normal PTH values are 150 to 300 pg/mL. During treatment with an active vitamin D sterol, levels of calcium, phosphorus, and serum PTH must be monitored and managed separately, depending on values.

130. D: If after initiation of calcitriol treatment for elevated PTH level, the patient's calcium level is 10.5 mg/dL, the appropriate response is to hold the calcitriol, as the level is greater than 10.2 mg/dL. High levels of calcium are associated with vascular calcification and increased mortality rates, especially if levels are greater than 12 mg/dL. Levels lower than 7 mg/dL also increase risks. The optimal level for patients is 9 to 12 mg/dL, but giving calcitriol at levels greater than 10.2 mg/dL may cause the level to increase over 12 mg/dL.

131. C: The statement by a patient on hemodialysis that most suggests that the patient may need a referral for psychological counseling is: "Some days I wish I didn't even wake up." Discontent with hemodialysis is common, and expressing those feelings can be helpful for patients. However, many patients become less adherent over time and many develop depression, so it is important to listen carefully for indications of depression or suicidal ideation and to actively question the patient about thoughts of suicide.

Section Description: Independent Questions, Group 3

132. A: If a female patient with CAPD has become increasingly withdrawn and is reluctant to be seen in public unless wearing a large coat, the patient is most likely experiencing body image disturbance. This is common because of abdominal distention and weight gain associated with CAPD. Additionally, lifestyle changes that are required to accommodate CAPD can challenge a patient's perception of self. Some patients may benefit from a fashion consultation to help them pick appropriate clothing that is stylish and flattering.

133. D: Considering the peritoneal equilibrium test (PET), patients categorized as high transporters would be expected to have the highest 4-hour dialysate to plasma creatinine, urea, and sodium (D/PCr, PUr, and PNa) values, usually because of large and effective peritoneal surface area and/or highly permeable membrane. However, dialysate glucose also diffuses quickly into the blood for the same reasons, resulting in low 4-hour dialysate to dialysate zero glucose values (D/D_0G). High transporters also tend to have higher loss of protein and serum albumin.

134. A: If a patient with CAPD has decreased effluent volumes of dialysate and increased weight gain without peripheral edema, and physical examination shows an asymmetric protuberant abdomen, the most likely cause is abdominal wall leak. The weight gain occurs as the fluid builds up in the abdominal wall tissues. The patient should stand during examination of the abdomen because asymmetry is more readily identified in this position. Abdominal wall leaks may result from poor surgical technique. The patient may need to convert to day dry APD or hemodialysis until the defect in the wall heals.

135. A: If a patient with CAPD has resorted to increasingly frequent use of more hypertonic glucose dialysate in order to prevent fluid overload and achieve target weight, the initial intervention should be to decrease sodium and fluid intake. While increasing hypertonicity can help to control fluid balance, it also increases serum glucose and can lead to weight gain, a common finding in patients with CAPD. Additionally, if the patient has gained body weight (as opposed to fluid), then the baseline target weight may need to be adjusted.

136. D: Potassium and uremic solutes diffuse from peritoneal capillary blood into peritoneal fluid during peritoneal dialysis while glucose and lactate or bicarbonate as well as calcium and magnesium diffuse in the opposite direction, from the dialysate into the capillary blood. Some potassium is also released from the peritoneal lining during dialysis. Potassium is commonly added to dialysate to compensate for the loss that occurs during treatment. Patients should be advised to eat foods high in potassium (3000 to 4000 mg/day is recommended).

137. B: Amino acid–based solution for peritoneal dialysis is indicated for nutritionally compromised patients and is essentially absorbed by the end of a 4- to 6-hour dwell. Amino acid–based solutions can only be used once per day as more frequent use may result in acidosis and increased blood urea. Amino acid–based solution is more effective with oral intake of adequate

calories, which is needed for protein synthesis. If a patient has poor intake of food, then the amino acid–based solution may be administered with glucose.

138. B: An upper chest presternal exit site for peritoneal dialysis may be indicated for patients who are morbidly obese. Presternal exit sites may also be used with patients who have an existing stoma as well as those who have a history of tunnel infection and those who are incontinent and wear adult diapers, resulting in increased risk of infection. Some advantages include the ability to take a tub bath and decreased irritation from clothing. The site also has less movement, so the catheter is more stable.

139. D: Mixing aminoglycosides (such as gentamicin, amikacin, netilmicin, paromomycin, and tobramycin) in the same dialysis solution bag with penicillins (a beta-lactam) is contraindicated because the drugs are incompatible. The penicillin may react with the aminoglycoside and interfere with the action of the aminoglycoside, rendering it less effective. Additionally, kidney disease may exacerbate this reaction. Antibiotics that can be mixed with penicillins include vancomycin and cephalosporins, such as cefazolin and ceftazidime.

140. D: Vancomycin is stable in dialysate stored at room temperature for up to 28 days; however, high ambient temperatures may render the antibiotic unstable earlier. Gentamicin (an aminoglycoside) is stable at room temperature for 14 days; if the solution contains heparin, this reduces the duration. Cefazolin (a cephalosporin) is stable at room temperature for 8 days and under refrigeration for 14 days, while ceftazidime (another cephalosporin) is stable for only 4 days at room temperature and 7 days if refrigerated.

141. B: If a patient with peritoneal dialysis is receiving intraperitoneal fluconazole for fungal peritonitis and begins to experience hallucinations and exhibit paranoid behavior, the nurse should suspect an overdose of the medication. Fungal peritonitis is often related to improper techniques for peritoneal dialysis, but fungal peritonitis can also occur secondary to antibiotic therapy. Most fungal peritonitis is caused by *Candida* spp. If fungi are found along with a bacterial infection, prognosis is poor because response to therapy is decreased.

142. B: If a patient on peritoneal dialysis tells the nurse that one of the employees at his company has offered to give him a kidney in exchange for $100,000, the nurse should advise the patient that it is illegal to buy or sell an organ. The patient could encounter both criminal and civil penalties, especially if the employee later claims coercion or suffers adverse effects. Additionally, the patient may be subjected to blackmail because of the illegal nature of the transaction.

Section Description: Woods Case Questions

143. D: The most common cause of acute kidney injury (AKI) in critically ill patients, especially elderly patients, is sepsis. Sepsis results in hemodynamic instability and hypoperfusion. Therefore, the first-line treatment is fluid resuscitation with intravenous fluids. However, because of increased vascular permeability resulting from inflammation, the fluid may move into the interstitial (third) space. Vasopressors are often used to combat hypotension, but they may also increase vascular resistance in the kidney microvasculature.

144. A: In a patient with AKI, if ECG telemetry shows peaked T waves and widening of the QRS interval (signs that may lead to ventricular tachycardia or fibrillation), these changes may be indicative of hyperkalemia. Other indications of hyperkalemia (>4.5 mEq/L) are irritability, anxiety,

nausea and vomiting, weakness, abdominal cramping, and numbness and tingling of the fingertips and around the mouth. With AKI, levels may increase to ≥6 mEq/L in a short period of time.

145. C: If a patient with acute renal failure has increasing peripheral edema and pulmonary congestion with decreased urinary output, the medication of choice is likely a loop diuretic, such as furosemide. Studies indicate that loop diuretics do not improve outcomes for patients who are severely ill with AKI; however, the diuretics increase urinary output and may relieve edema and pulmonary congestion in patients with heart failure, so they are frequently prescribed.

146. B: If a patient with AKI and anuria has a potassium level that has increased from 4.5 to 6 mmol/L in a short time, the most likely temporary emergent treatment is insulin (10 units regular) and glucose (50 mL of dextrose 50% solution) per infusion because this causes the potassium to move from the serum and into the cells. Diuretics may be given to decrease potassium but only if the patient is producing adequate urine. Sodium polystyrene sulfonate (Kayexalate) or dialysis may be used as permanent methods to reduce potassium levels.

147. B: In a patient with acute kidney injury, if the serum creatinine (a byproduct of muscle metabolism) increases from 0.75 to 1.5 mg/dL, the nurse expects that the GFR will decrease by 50%. Normal creatinine ranges from 0.5 to 1.2 mg/dL (45 to 107 micromol/L). The potential critical value is greater than 7.4 mg/dL in nondialytic patients. Chronic renal insufficiency occurs with creatinine of 1.5 to 3 mg/dL with renal failure present at greater than 3 mg/dL.

Section Description: Washington Case Questions

148. D: When instructing a patient in the use of a preattached double bag system for peritoneal dialysis, the patient should be advised to flush 100 mL of dialysate from the fill bag to the drainage bag before filling the peritoneal cavity. This procedure removes residual air from the tubing. The fill bag (afferent limb of the Y) is opened by breaking a frangible device in the tubing. After flushing, the efferent limb is clamped and the afferent limb unclamped.

149. A: The primary advantage of a 2-compartment peritoneal dialysis solution bag is to allow delivery at normal pH. Standard lactate-based dialysate has a pH of 5.5 because heat sterilization of glucose generates fewer glucose degradation products at low pH; however, low pH may also cause pain during inflow. Additionally, low pH may impair both the immune response to bacteria and the peritoneal membrane, so with 2-compartment dialysate, the smaller portion that contains glucose is heated at a very low pH and the other portion at a higher pH and then the fluids are mixed before administration to achieve normal pH.

150. A: The 3 transport processes that occur at the same time during the course of peritoneal dialysis are as follows:
   1. Diffusion: Solutes move from the dialysate into the capillary blood and from the capillary blood into the dialysate depending various factors, including the concentration gradient and molecular weight of solutes.
   2. Ultrafiltration: Occurs because of the presence of an osmotic agent, such as glucose.
   3. Absorption: Fluid is absorbed via lymphatics and the parietal peritoneum.

Section Description: Lee Case Questions

151. D: If a patient is referred to physical therapy for exercises to mature a fistula that was created 1 week earlier in the lower arm, the exercises likely include ball squeeze to slow blood return and

dilate the fistula. Other exercises include squeezing and opening a clothespin for 5 minutes or touching fingers to thumb tip. Exercises are done for 5 to 10 minutes up to 6 times daily. Exercises for fistulas in the upper arm include hammer and bicep curls using light weights, 1 to 3 pounds.

152. C: During the first week of treatment with a new AV fistula, the initial needle size is usually 17-gauge because a larger needle may damage the fistula, especially if it infiltrates. The initial flow rate is also kept low at 200 to 250 mL/min. The physician will determine when the needle size and flow rate are to increase, based on feedback provided by cannulators. New AV fistula should never be cannulated by inexperienced staff.

153. B: With an AV fistula, cannulation should be done at an angle of 25° to 35°. Improperly cannulating an AV fistula may result in pain and anxiety on the part of the patient and premature failure of the access site. AV grafts should be cannulated at an angle of 45°. Steps to cannulation include inspecting the AV site and arm for discoloration or breaks in the skin, palpating for a thrill, and auscultating to assess the flow of blood and the bruit.

154. D: According to the "Rule of 6s," an AV fistula is considered successful if it is 0.6 cm wide, is positioned less than 0.6 cm below the skin surface, and has a blood flow rate of at least 600 mL/min as verified by ultrasound. The AV fistula if the recommended access for hemodialysis because it is the longest lasting and tends to have a lower risk of blood clotting. Use of the patient's own vessels is preferred. One problem with the AV fistula is that it can take 1 to 4 months to mature, during which an alternate access is required.

155. A: If an infection occurs in an arteriovenous graft, the patient is at increased risk of hemorrhage because the infection may cause the graft material to disintegrate. Grafts may be biologic, semi-biologic, or prosthetic (most commonly made from Teflon or fabric) and are implanted to form an anastomosis between a vein and artery. Arteriovenous grafts pose a greater risk of infection than arteriovenous fistulas and have a shorter life span, typically 2 to 3 years.

Case Description: Shaw Case Questions

156. D: For a patient receiving APD with most dialysis occurring during the night, the best time to take a plasma sample to determine the urea level is mid-afternoon because this is usually in the middle of the non-cycling period. For patients receiving APD, the urea level is usually lowest in the early morning at the end of cycling and highest in the evening before cycling. For patients receiving CAPD, the urea levels stay fairly stable because dialysis is continuous, so serum can be obtained at any time during the day.

157. B: With APD, icodextrin may be used rather than glucose solution for the long day dwell. Icodextrin is a polyglucose solution that induces ultrafiltration and is absorbed by the lymphatics at a slower rate than glucose, making it best suited for long dwells, such as the long nocturnal dwell with CAPD and the long daytime dwell with APD. It is not used for short dwells because it is not more effective than glucose and is more costly. Icodextrin is generally restricted to only 1 long dwell daily.

158. C: With APD, the patient should expect to spend 8 to 10 nighttime hours cycling. The number of cycles per night may vary from 3 to 10 with various dwell times, usually beginning at about 10 PM and continuing until about 7 AM. A variety of different patterns may be used with APD:
- Day dry: night cycles with no daytime dwell.
- Long day dwell: night cycles with long daytime dwell.

- Morning dwell: night cycles with morning dwell until noon.
- Evening dwell: night cycles with evening dwell from 5 to 10 PM.

Section Description: Rule Case Questions

159. B: Hemolytic uremic syndrome (HUS), a complication of *E. coli* (O157:H7) infection, is characterized by the triad of (1) acute renal failure, (2) microangiopathic hemolytic anemia, and (3) thrombocytopenia. HUS is most common in children younger than 5 years or older adults. Bacterial toxins from the *E. coli* enter the bloodstream from the intestines, causing damage to small vessels in the kidneys and sometimes other organs as well. Urinary output decreases as the diarrhea progresses.

160. D: Initial therapy for HUS usually includes intravenous fluids to maintain fluid and electrolyte balance. Antibiotics should generally be avoided because they may stimulate the release of extra toxin; however, antibiotics may be necessary if the patient develops sepsis. Antimotility agents increase the risk that the *E. coli* infection will progress to HUS and they should be avoided as well. Plasmapheresis may be used to remove antibodies from the blood. ACE inhibitors may help prevent permanent kidney damage.

161. A: With HUS, the part of the kidney that is damaged is the glomeruli. Toxins destroy platelets and clotting time increases. Red blood cells fragment when they flow through areas of thrombi. The glomeruli are damaged when they become obstructed with damaged platelets and red blood cells, interfering with the kidneys' ability to filter waste products. About half of the patients with HUS progress to acute kidney failure and some may require ongoing dialysis or kidney transplant. About a third of those who develop kidney failure have delayed abnormalities of kidney function later in life.

Section Description: Branch Case Study

162. B: If a hospitalized patient is newly diagnosed with kidney failure and in need of peritoneal dialysis, but the patient has little income, inadequate insurance, and little social support, the best initial referral is to a social worker who can assess the patient's resources and needs. The social worker can advise the patient about eligibility for Medicaid and other services in the community and make appropriate referrals to enable the patient to manage the condition.

163. A: If, when teaching a patient to manage CAPD, the nurse is concerned that the patient may lack the manual dexterity needed to manage the procedure, the best professional to assess this is an occupational therapist. The occupational therapist can assess the patient's ability to carry out needed tasks and can determine if modifications or assistive devices are appropriate to help the patient remain independent in carrying out treatment. The occupational therapist can customize interventions to meet the patient's needs.

164. B: The statement by a patient undergoing peritoneal dialysis indicating the need for referral to a nutritionist is: "I can have all of the salt I want in my diet." While there has been some debate about the value of sodium restriction to prevent cardiovascular disease, and increasing the glucose hypertonicity of dialysate can help to remove excess fluids, doing so routinely can lead to increased serum glucose, damage to the peritoneal membrane, weight gain, and hyperlipidemia, so patients need to limit sodium intake, ideally to about 1.5 g/day.

165. B: If a 40-year-old patient using CAPD for ESKD is concerned about losing employment because of the inability to carry out all aspects of the job, the best initial solution for the patient is likely to ask for accommodation per the ADA. It is better for patients to discuss their needs with employers to determine if the workload or procedures can be modified than to try to do work they are physically unable to do or to put themselves in a position to be fired.

166. B: If a patient receiving peritoneal dialysis (PD) for ESKD frequently exhibits denial regarding physical decline but adheres closely to treatment regimens and remains cheerful, the best response to this patient's denial is to allow the patient to use denial. Some degree of denial can help patients to cope with situations that may otherwise cause severe anxiety. While extreme denial may result in nonadherence, the fact that this patient adheres closely to treatment suggests the patient has some degree of realistic perception.

Section Description: Anders Case Questions

167. C: A patient with diabetes mellitus (either type 1 or type 2) and chronic kidney disease should generally have a target HbA$_{1c}$ of less than 7%, but the A$_{1c}$ may be individualized for the patient with type 2 diabetes. Additionally, KDIGO guidelines suggest that the target may need to be adjusted upward for patients who tend to be hypoglycemic or have multiple comorbidities. Good glycemic control can slow progression of kidney disease.

168. C: In a diabetic patient with chronic kidney failure, glycosuria is unreliable as an estimation of hyperglycemia because the damaged nephrons may be inconsistent in excreting excess glucose. Normally, urine does not contain glucose; however, if there is an excess load of glucose, it may not all be reabsorbed. With normal kidney function, glycosuria usually occurs when serum glucose levels are greater than 180 mg/dL, but with kidney failure, this may vary widely.

169. B: When teaching a patient with chronic kidney disease about dietary restrictions, the nurse should generally advise the patient to limit daily protein intake to 0.8 g/kg. There remains some controversy about the benefit of protein restrictions, and restriction below this level is usually not recommended. Evidence has been shown that limiting protein may reduce the progression of chronic kidney disease. Patients who are malnourished may need to have some additional protein.

170. C: Patients with chronic kidney disease often develop normocytic, normochromic anemia because production within the bone marrow is not impaired, but as the erythropoietin level falls, it does not adequately stimulate production of red blood cells. However, patients may also develop other types of anemia because of nutritional deficiencies, more rapid hemolysis of red blood cells, GI bleeding, blood sampling, and hemodialysis. Additionally, elevated parathyroid hormone levels may inhibit erythropoiesis and shorten survival of red blood cells.

171. B: According to KDIGO guidelines, treatment with an erythropoiesis-stimulating agent (ESA) for anemia associated with chronic kidney disease should not be initiated until the hemoglobin level falls to less than 10 g/dL. Anemia tends to worsen as the kidneys fail, resulting in anemia because of deficiency of erythropoietin or iron; however, using an ESA to increase the hemoglobin level to 13 g/dL shows no benefit and may increase risk of complications and has no effect on the progression of kidney disease, so only partial correction is generally done.

172. C: As chronic kidney disease progresses, the endocrinologic change that can result in higher risk of fractures is hyperparathyroidism. As kidney function declines, less vitamin D is converted to its active form, so less calcium is absorbed, resulting in hypocalcemia. As a compensatory measure,

the parathyroid gland secretes increased amounts of parathyroid hormone (PTH) to stimulate demineralization and release increased amounts of the calcium and phosphate from the bones, resulting in weakened bony matrix.

173. C: Kidney failure is generally considered inevitable when loss of kidney function reaches 50% to 60%. Patients may stabilize if treatment is able to reverse some of the kidney damage before patients lose 40% to 50% of kidney function. As nephrons are lost, hyperfiltration occurs in the remaining glomeruli in order to increase the GFR, but this causes stress and damage to the glomeruli. If this downward spiral continues, the patient will develop ESKD.

174. D: A patient with chronic kidney disease must have dialysis or transplantation in order to survive when kidney function falls below 10% to 15%, the indication for ESKD (stage 5 kidney failure). Prior to this, CKD may be managed with some combination of fluid restriction, dietary sodium restriction, and medications (such as ARBs, phosphate binders, and diuretics). The patient's quality of life may gradually deteriorate as the GFR falls because of increasing physical limitations and complications.

175. A: Dialysis is usually started when a patient with uremia has a GFR (MDRD equation) of <15 mL/min/1.73 m². Stages of chronic kidney disease are as follows:
1. GRF remains relatively normal (≥90 mL/min/1.73 m²)
2. GFR decreasing (60 to 89 mL/min/1.73 m²) with mild kidney damage and focus on assessing progression
3. GFR further decreases (30 to 59 mL/min/1.73 m²) with moderate kidney damage and focus on evaluating and treating complications
4. GFR decreases (15 to 29 mL/min/1.73 m²) with severe kidney damage and focus on preparing for dialysis
5. Kidney failure with GRF <15 mL/min/1.73 m² and a candidate for dialysis and/or kidney transplant

Secret Key #1 - Time is Your Greatest Enemy

Pace Yourself

Wear a watch. At the beginning of the test, check the time (or start a chronometer on your watch to count the minutes), and check the time after every few questions to make sure you are "on schedule."

If you are forced to speed up, do it efficiently. Usually one or more answer choices can be eliminated without too much difficulty. Above all, don't panic. Don't speed up and just begin guessing at random choices. By pacing yourself, and continually monitoring your progress against your watch, you will always know exactly how far ahead or behind you are with your available time. If you find that you are one minute behind on the test, don't skip one question without spending any time on it, just to catch back up. Take 15 fewer seconds on the next four questions, and after four questions you'll have caught back up. Once you catch back up, you can continue working each problem at your normal pace.

Furthermore, don't dwell on the problems that you were rushed on. If a problem was taking up too much time and you made a hurried guess, it must be difficult. The difficult questions are the ones you are most likely to miss anyway, so it isn't a big loss. It is better to end with more time than you need than to run out of time.

Lastly, sometimes it is beneficial to slow down if you are constantly getting ahead of time. You are always more likely to catch a careless mistake by working more slowly than quickly, and among very high-scoring test takers (those who are likely to have lots of time left over), careless errors affect the score more than mastery of material.

Secret Key #2 - Guessing is not Guesswork

You probably know that guessing is a good idea. Unlike other standardized tests, there is no penalty for getting a wrong answer. Even if you have no idea about a question, you still have a 20-25% chance of getting it right.

Most test takers do not understand the impact that proper guessing can have on their score. Unless you score extremely high, guessing will significantly contribute to your final score.

Monkeys Take the Test

What most test takers don't realize is that to insure that 20-25% chance, you have to guess randomly. If you put 20 monkeys in a room to take this test, assuming they answered once per question and behaved themselves, on average they would get 20-25% of the questions correct. Put 20 test takers in the room, and the average will be much lower among guessed questions. Why?
　　1. The test writers intentionally write deceptive answer choices that "look" right. A test taker has no idea about a question, so he picks the "best looking" answer, which is often wrong.

The monkey has no idea what looks good and what doesn't, so it will consistently be right about 20-25% of the time.
2. Test takers will eliminate answer choices from the guessing pool based on a hunch or intuition. Simple but correct answers often get excluded, leaving a 0% chance of being correct. The monkey has no clue, and often gets lucky with the best choice.

This is why the process of elimination endorsed by most test courses is flawed and detrimental to your performance. Test takers don't guess; they make an ignorant stab in the dark that is usually worse than random.

$5 Challenge

Let me introduce one of the most valuable ideas of this course—the $5 challenge:

You only mark your "best guess" if you are willing to bet $5 on it.
You only eliminate choices from guessing if you are willing to bet $5 on it.

Why $5? Five dollars is an amount of money that is small yet not insignificant, and can really add up fast (20 questions could cost you $100). Likewise, each answer choice on one question of the test will have a small impact on your overall score, but it can really add up to a lot of points in the end.

The process of elimination IS valuable. The following shows your chance of guessing it right:

If you eliminate wrong answer choices until only this many remain:	Chance of getting it correct:
1	100%
2	50%
3	33%

However, if you accidentally eliminate the right answer or go on a hunch for an incorrect answer, your chances drop dramatically—to 0%. By guessing among all the answer choices, you are GUARANTEED to have a shot at the right answer.

That's why the $5 test is so valuable. If you give up the advantage and safety of a pure guess, it had better be worth the risk.

What we still haven't covered is how to be sure that whatever guess you make is truly random. Here's the easiest way:

Always pick the first answer choice among those remaining.

Such a technique means that you have decided, **before you see a single test question**, exactly how you are going to guess, and since the order of choices tells you nothing about which one is correct, this guessing technique is perfectly random.

This section is not meant to scare you away from making educated guesses or eliminating choices; you just need to define when a choice is worth eliminating. The $5 test, along with a pre-defined random guessing strategy, is the best way to make sure you reap all of the benefits of guessing.

Secret Key #3 - Practice Smarter, Not Harder

Many test takers delay the test preparation process because they dread the awful amounts of practice time they think necessary to succeed on the test. We have refined an effective method that will take you only a fraction of the time.

There are a number of "obstacles" in the path to success. Among these are answering questions, finishing in time, and mastering test-taking strategies. All must be executed on the day of the test at peak performance, or your score will suffer. The test is a mental marathon that has a large impact on your future.

Just like a marathon runner, it is important to work your way up to the full challenge. So first you just worry about questions, and then time, and finally strategy:

Success Strategy

1. Find a good source for practice tests.
2. If you are willing to make a larger time investment, consider using more than one study guide. Often the different approaches of multiple authors will help you "get" difficult concepts.
3. Take a practice test with no time constraints, with all study helps, "open book." Take your time with questions and focus on applying strategies.
4. Take a practice test with time constraints, with all guides, "open book."
5. Take a final practice test without open material and with time limits.

If you have time to take more practice tests, just repeat step 5. By gradually exposing yourself to the full rigors of the test environment, you will condition your mind to the stress of test day and maximize your success.

Secret Key #4 - Prepare, Don't Procrastinate

Let me state an obvious fact: if you take the test three times, you will probably get three different scores. This is due to the way you feel on test day, the level of preparedness you have, and the version of the test you see. Despite the test writers' claims to the contrary, some versions of the test WILL be easier for you than others.

Since your future depends so much on your score, you should maximize your chances of success. In order to maximize the likelihood of success, you've got to prepare in advance. This means taking practice tests and spending time learning the information and test taking strategies you will need to succeed.

Never go take the actual test as a "practice" test, expecting that you can just take it again if you need to. Take all the practice tests you can on your own, but when you go to take the official test, be prepared, be focused, and do your best the first time!

Secret Key #5 - Test Yourself

Everyone knows that time is money. There is no need to spend too much of your time or too little of your time preparing for the test. You should only spend as much of your precious time preparing as is necessary for you to get the score you need.

Once you have taken a practice test under real conditions of time constraints, then you will know if you are ready for the test or not.

If you have scored extremely high the first time that you take the practice test, then there is not much point in spending countless hours studying. You are already there.

Benchmark your abilities by retaking practice tests and seeing how much you have improved. Once you consistently score high enough to guarantee success, then you are ready.

If you have scored well below where you need, then knuckle down and begin studying in earnest. Check your improvement regularly through the use of practice tests under real conditions. Above all, don't worry, panic, or give up. The key is perseverance!

Then, when you go to take the test, remain confident and remember how well you did on the practice tests. If you can score high enough on a practice test, then you can do the same on the real thing.

General Strategies

The most important thing you can do is to ignore your fears and jump into the test immediately. Do not be overwhelmed by any strange-sounding terms. You have to jump into the test like jumping into a pool—all at once is the easiest way.

Make Predictions

As you read and understand the question, try to guess what the answer will be. Remember that several of the answer choices are wrong, and once you begin reading them, your mind will immediately become cluttered with answer choices designed to throw you off. Your mind is typically the most focused immediately after you have read the question and digested its contents. If you can, try to predict what the correct answer will be. You may be surprised at what you can predict.

Quickly scan the choices and see if your prediction is in the listed answer choices. If it is, then you can be quite confident that you have the right answer. It still won't hurt to check the other answer choices, but most of the time, you've got it!

Answer the Question

It may seem obvious to only pick answer choices that answer the question, but the test writers can create some excellent answer choices that are wrong. Don't pick an answer just because it sounds right, or you believe it to be true. It MUST answer the question. Once you've made your selection, always go back and check it against the question and make sure that you didn't misread the question and that the answer choice does answer the question posed.

Benchmark

After you read the first answer choice, decide if you think it sounds correct or not. If it doesn't, move on to the next answer choice. If it does, mentally mark that answer choice. This doesn't mean that you've definitely selected it as your answer choice, it just means that it's the best you've seen thus far. Go ahead and read the next choice. If the next choice is worse than the one you've already selected, keep going to the next answer choice. If the next choice is better than the choice you've already selected, mentally mark the new answer choice as your best guess.

The first answer choice that you select becomes your standard. Every other answer choice must be benchmarked against that standard. That choice is correct until proven otherwise by another answer choice beating it out. Once you've decided that no other answer choice seems as good, do one final check to ensure that your answer choice answers the question posed.

Valid Information

Don't discount any of the information provided in the question. Every piece of information may be necessary to determine the correct answer. None of the information in the question is there to throw you off (while the answer choices will certainly have information to throw you off). If two seemingly unrelated topics are discussed, don't ignore either. You can be confident there is a relationship, or it wouldn't be included in the question, and you are probably going to have to determine what is that relationship to find the answer.

Avoid "Fact Traps"

Don't get distracted by a choice that is factually true. Your search is for the answer that answers the question. Stay focused and don't fall for an answer that is true but irrelevant. Always go back to the question and make sure you're choosing an answer that actually answers the question and is not just a true statement. An answer can be factually correct, but it MUST answer the question asked. Additionally, two answers can both be seemingly correct, so be sure to read all of the answer choices, and make sure that you get the one that BEST answers the question.

Milk the Question

Some of the questions may throw you completely off. They might deal with a subject you have not been exposed to, or one that you haven't reviewed in years. While your lack of knowledge about the subject will be a hindrance, the question itself can give you many clues that will help you find the correct answer. Read the question carefully and look for clues. Watch particularly for adjectives and nouns describing difficult terms or words that you don't recognize. Regardless of whether you completely understand a word or not, replacing it with a synonym, either provided or one you more familiar with, may help you to understand what the questions are asking. Rather than wracking your mind about specific detailed information concerning a difficult term or word, try to use mental substitutes that are easier to understand.

The Trap of Familiarity

Don't just choose a word because you recognize it. On difficult questions, you may not recognize a number of words in the answer choices. The test writers don't put "make-believe" words on the test, so don't think that just because you only recognize all the words in one answer choice that that answer choice must be correct. If you only recognize words in one answer choice, then focus on that one. Is it correct? Try your best to determine if it is correct. If it is, that's great. If not, eliminate it. Each word and answer choice you eliminate increases your chances of getting the question correct, even if you then have to guess among the unfamiliar choices.

Eliminate Answers

Eliminate choices as soon as you realize they are wrong. But be careful! Make sure you consider all of the possible answer choices. Just because one appears right, doesn't mean that the next one won't be even better! The test writers will usually put more than one good answer choice for every question, so read all of them. Don't worry if you are stuck between two that seem right. By getting down to just two remaining possible choices, your odds are now 50/50. Rather than wasting too much time, play the odds. You are guessing, but guessing wisely because you've been able to knock out some of the answer choices that you know are wrong. If you are eliminating choices and realize that the last answer choice you are left with is also obviously wrong, don't panic. Start over and consider each choice again. There may easily be something that you missed the first time and will realize on the second pass.

Tough Questions

If you are stumped on a problem or it appears too hard or too difficult, don't waste time. Move on! Remember though, if you can quickly check for obviously incorrect answer choices, your chances of guessing correctly are greatly improved. Before you completely give up, at least try to knock out a couple of possible answers. Eliminate what you can and then guess at the remaining answer choices before moving on.

Brainstorm

If you get stuck on a difficult question, spend a few seconds quickly brainstorming. Run through the complete list of possible answer choices. Look at each choice and ask yourself, "Could this answer the question satisfactorily?" Go through each answer choice and consider it independently of the others. By systematically going through all possibilities, you may find something that you would otherwise overlook. Remember though that when you get stuck, it's important to try to keep moving.

Read Carefully

Understand the problem. Read the question and answer choices carefully. Don't miss the question because you misread the terms. You have plenty of time to read each question thoroughly and make sure you understand what is being asked. Yet a happy medium must be attained, so don't waste too much time. You must read carefully, but efficiently.

Face Value

When in doubt, use common sense. Always accept the situation in the problem at face value. Don't read too much into it. These problems will not require you to make huge leaps of logic. The test writers aren't trying to throw you off with a cheap trick. If you have to go beyond creativity and make a leap of logic in order to have an answer choice answer the question, then you should look at the other answer choices. Don't overcomplicate the problem by creating theoretical relationships or explanations that will warp time or space. These are normal problems rooted in reality. It's just that the applicable relationship or explanation may not be readily apparent and you have to figure things out. Use your common sense to interpret anything that isn't clear.

Prefixes

If you're having trouble with a word in the question or answer choices, try dissecting it. Take advantage of every clue that the word might include. Prefixes and suffixes can be a huge help. Usually they allow you to determine a basic meaning. Pre- means before, post- means after, pro - is positive, de- is negative. From these prefixes and suffixes, you can get an idea of the general meaning of the word and try to put it into context. Beware though of any traps. Just because con- is the opposite of pro-, doesn't necessarily mean congress is the opposite of progress!

Hedge Phrases

Watch out for critical hedge phrases, led off with words such as "likely," "may," "can," "sometimes," "often," "almost," "mostly," "usually," "generally," "rarely," and "sometimes." Question writers insert these hedge phrases to cover every possibility. Often an answer choice will be wrong simply because it leaves no room for exception. Unless the situation calls for them, avoid answer choices that have definitive words like "exactly," and "always."

Switchback Words

Stay alert for "switchbacks." These are the words and phrases frequently used to alert you to shifts in thought. The most common switchback word is "but." Others include "although," "however," "nevertheless," "on the other hand," "even though," "while," "in spite of," "despite," and "regardless of."

New Information

Correct answer choices will rarely have completely new information included. Answer choices typically are straightforward reflections of the material asked about and will directly relate to the question. If a new piece of information is included in an answer choice that doesn't even seem to relate to the topic being asked about, then that answer choice is likely incorrect. All of the information needed to answer the question is usually provided for you in the question. You should not have to make guesses that are unsupported or choose answer choices that require unknown information that cannot be reasoned from what is given.

Time Management

On technical questions, don't get lost on the technical terms. Don't spend too much time on any one question. If you don't know what a term means, then odds are you aren't going to get much further since you don't have a dictionary. You should be able to immediately recognize whether or not you know a term. If you don't, work with the other clues that you have—the other answer choices and terms provided—but don't waste too much time trying to figure out a difficult term that you don't know.

Contextual Clues

Look for contextual clues. An answer can be right but not the correct answer. The contextual clues will help you find the answer that is most right and is correct. Understand the context in which a phrase or statement is made. This will help you make important distinctions.

Don't Panic

Panicking will not answer any questions for you; therefore, it isn't helpful. When you first see the question, if your mind goes blank, take a deep breath. Force yourself to mechanically go through the steps of solving the problem using the strategies you've learned.

Pace Yourself

Don't get clock fever. It's easy to be overwhelmed when you're looking at a page full of questions, your mind is full of random thoughts and feeling confused, and the clock is ticking down faster than you would like. Calm down and maintain the pace that you have set for yourself. As long as you are on track by monitoring your pace, you are guaranteed to have enough time for yourself. When you get to the last few minutes of the test, it may seem like you won't have enough time left, but if you only have as many questions as you should have left at that point, then you're right on track!

Answer Selection

The best way to pick an answer choice is to eliminate all of those that are wrong, until only one is left and confirm that is the correct answer. Sometimes though, an answer choice may immediately look right. Be careful! Take a second to make sure that the other choices are not equally obvious. Don't make a hasty mistake. There are only two times that you should stop before checking other answers. First is when you are positive that the answer choice you have selected is correct. Second is when time is almost out and you have to make a quick guess!

Check Your Work

Since you will probably not know every term listed and the answer to every question, it is important that you get credit for the ones that you do know. Don't miss any questions through careless mistakes. If at all possible, try to take a second to look back over your answer selection and make sure you've selected the correct answer choice and haven't made a costly careless mistake (such as marking an answer choice that you didn't mean to mark). The time it takes for this quick double check should more than pay for itself in caught mistakes.

Beware of Directly Quoted Answers

Sometimes an answer choice will repeat word for word a portion of the question or reference section. However, beware of such exact duplication. It may be a trap! More than likely, the correct choice will paraphrase or summarize a point, rather than being exactly the same wording.

Slang

Scientific sounding answers are better than slang ones. An answer choice that begins "To compare the outcomes..." is much more likely to be correct than one that begins "Because some people insisted..."

Extreme Statements

Avoid wild answers that throw out highly controversial ideas that are proclaimed as established fact. An answer choice that states the "process should used in certain situations, if..." is much more likely to be correct than one that states the "process should be discontinued completely." The first is a calm rational statement and doesn't even make a definitive, uncompromising stance, using a hedge word "if" to provide wiggle room, whereas the second choice is a radical idea and far more extreme.

Answer Choice Families

When you have two or more answer choices that are direct opposites or parallels, one of them is usually the correct answer. For instance, if one answer choice states "x increases" and another answer choice states "x decreases" or "y increases," then those two or three answer choices are very similar in construction and fall into the same family of answer choices. A family of answer choices consists of two or three answer choices, very similar in construction, but often with directly opposite meanings. Usually the correct answer choice will be in that family of answer choices. The "odd man out" or answer choice that doesn't seem to fit the parallel construction of the other answer choices is more likely to be incorrect.

Special Report: How to Overcome Test Anxiety

The very nature of tests caters to some level of anxiety, nervousness, or tension, just as we feel for any important event that occurs in our lives. A little bit of anxiety or nervousness can be a good thing. It helps us with motivation, and makes achievement just that much sweeter. However, too much anxiety can be a problem, especially if it hinders our ability to function and perform.

"Test anxiety," is the term that refers to the emotional reactions that some test-takers experience when faced with a test or exam. Having a fear of testing and exams is based upon a rational fear, since the test-taker's performance can shape the course of an academic career. Nevertheless, experiencing excessive fear of examinations will only interfere with the test-taker's ability to perform and chance to be successful.

There are a large variety of causes that can contribute to the development and sensation of test anxiety. These include, but are not limited to, lack of preparation and worrying about issues surrounding the test.

Lack of Preparation

Lack of preparation can be identified by the following behaviors or situations:

Not scheduling enough time to study, and therefore cramming the night before the test or exam
Managing time poorly, to create the sensation that there is not enough time to do everything
Failing to organize the text information in advance, so that the study material consists of the entire text and not simply the pertinent information
Poor overall studying habits

Worrying, on the other hand, can be related to both the test taker, or many other factors around him/her that will be affected by the results of the test. These include worrying about:

Previous performances on similar exams, or exams in general
How friends and other students are achieving
The negative consequences that will result from a poor grade or failure

There are three primary elements to test anxiety. Physical components, which involve the same typical bodily reactions as those to acute anxiety (to be discussed below). Emotional factors have to do with fear or panic. Mental or cognitive issues concerning attention spans and memory abilities.

Physical Signals

There are many different symptoms of test anxiety, and these are not limited to mental and emotional strain. Frequently there are a range of physical signals that will let a test taker know that he/she is suffering from test anxiety. These bodily changes can include the following:

Perspiring
Sweaty palms
Wet, trembling hands
Nausea
Dry mouth
A knot in the stomach
Headache
Faintness
Muscle tension
Aching shoulders, back and neck
Rapid heart beat
Feeling too hot/cold

To recognize the sensation of test anxiety, a test-taker should monitor him/herself for the following sensations:

The physical distress symptoms as listed above
Emotional sensitivity, expressing emotional feelings such as the need to cry or laugh too much, or a sensation of anger or helplessness
A decreased ability to think, causing the test-taker to blank out or have racing thoughts that are hard to organize or control.

Though most students will feel some level of anxiety when faced with a test or exam, the majority can cope with that anxiety and maintain it at a manageable level. However, those who cannot are faced with a very real and very serious condition, which can and should be controlled for the immeasurable benefit of this sufferer.

Naturally, these sensations lead to negative results for the testing experience. The most common effects of test anxiety have to do with nervousness and mental blocking.

Nervousness

Nervousness can appear in several different levels:

The test-taker's difficulty, or even inability to read and understand the questions on the test
The difficulty or inability to organize thoughts to a coherent form
The difficulty or inability to recall key words and concepts relating to the testing questions (especially essays)
The receipt of poor grades on a test, though the test material was well known by the test taker

Conversely, a person may also experience mental blocking, which involves:

Blanking out on test questions
Only remembering the correct answers to the questions when the test has already finished.

Fortunately for test anxiety sufferers, beating these feelings, to a large degree, has to do with proper preparation. When a test taker has a feeling of preparedness, then anxiety will be dramatically lessened.

The first step to resolving anxiety issues is to distinguish which of the two types of anxiety are being suffered. If the anxiety is a direct result of a lack of preparation, this should be considered a normal reaction, and the anxiety level (as opposed to the test results) shouldn't be anything to worry about. However, if, when adequately prepared, the test-taker still panics, blanks out, or seems to overreact, this is not a fully rational reaction. While this can be considered normal too, there are many ways to combat and overcome these effects.

Remember that anxiety cannot be entirely eliminated, however, there are ways to minimize it, to make the anxiety easier to manage. Preparation is one of the best ways to minimize test anxiety. Therefore the following techniques are wise in order to best fight off any anxiety that may want to build.

To begin with, try to avoid cramming before a test, whenever it is possible. By trying to memorize an entire term's worth of information in one day, you'll be shocking your system, and not giving yourself a very good chance to absorb the information. This is an easy path to anxiety, so for those who suffer from test anxiety, cramming should not even be considered an option.

Instead of cramming, work throughout the semester to combine all of the material which is presented throughout the semester, and work on it gradually as the course goes by, making sure to master the main concepts first, leaving minor details for a week or so before the test.

To study for the upcoming exam, be sure to pose questions that may be on the examination, to gauge the ability to answer them by integrating the ideas from your texts, notes and lectures, as well as any supplementary readings.

If it is truly impossible to cover all of the information that was covered in that particular term, concentrate on the most important portions, that can be covered very well. Learn these concepts as best as possible, so that when the test comes, a goal can be made to use these concepts as presentations of your knowledge.

In addition to study habits, changes in attitude are critical to beating a struggle with test anxiety. In fact, an improvement of the perspective over the entire test-taking experience can actually help a test taker to enjoy studying and therefore improve the overall experience. Be certain not to overemphasize the significance of the grade - know that the result of the test is neither a reflection of self worth, nor is it a measure of intelligence; one grade will not predict a person's future success.

To improve an overall testing outlook, the following steps should be tried:

Keeping in mind that the most reasonable expectation for taking a test is to expect to try to demonstrate as much of what you know as you possibly can.

Reminding ourselves that a test is only one test; this is not the only one, and there will be others.
The thought of thinking of oneself in an irrational, all-or-nothing term should be avoided at all costs.
A reward should be designated for after the test, so there's something to look forward to. Whether it be going to a movie, going out to eat, or simply visiting friends, schedule it in advance, and do it no matter what result is expected on the exam.

Test-takers should also keep in mind that the basics are some of the most important things, even beyond anti-anxiety techniques and studying. Never neglect the basic social, emotional and biological needs, in order to try to absorb information. In order to best achieve, these three factors must be held as just as important as the studying itself.

Study Steps

Remember the following important steps for studying:

Maintain healthy nutrition and exercise habits. Continue both your recreational activities and social pass times. These both contribute to your physical and emotional well being.
Be certain to get a good amount of sleep, especially the night before the test, because when you're overtired you are not able to perform to the best of your best ability.
Keep the studying pace to a moderate level by taking breaks when they are needed, and varying the work whenever possible, to keep the mind fresh instead of getting bored.
When enough studying has been done that all the material that can be learned has been learned, and the test taker is prepared for the test, stop studying and do something relaxing such as listening to music, watching a movie, or taking a warm bubble bath.

There are also many other techniques to minimize the uneasiness or apprehension that is experienced along with test anxiety before, during, or even after the examination. In fact, there are a great deal of things that can be done to stop anxiety from interfering with lifestyle and performance. Again, remember that anxiety will not be eliminated entirely, and it shouldn't be. Otherwise that "up" feeling for exams would not exist, and most of us depend on that sensation to perform better than usual. However, this anxiety has to be at a level that is manageable.

Of course, as we have just discussed, being prepared for the exam is half the battle right away. Attending all classes, finding out what knowledge will be expected on the exam, and knowing the exam schedules are easy steps to lowering anxiety. Keeping up with work will remove the need to cram, and efficient study habits will eliminate wasted time. Studying should be done in an ideal location for concentration, so that it is simple to become interested in the material and give it complete attention. A method such as SQ3R (Survey, Question, Read, Recite, Review) is a wonderful key to follow to make sure that the study habits are as effective as possible, especially in the case of learning from a textbook. Flashcards are great techniques for memorization. Learning to take good notes will mean that notes will be full of useful information, so that less sifting will need to be done to seek out what is pertinent for studying. Reviewing notes after class and then again on occasion will keep the information fresh in the mind. From notes that have been taken summary sheets and outlines can be made for simpler reviewing.

A study group can also be a very motivational and helpful place to study, as there will be a sharing of ideas, all of the minds can work together, to make sure that everyone understands, and the studying will be made more interesting because it will be a social occasion.

Basically, though, as long as the test-taker remains organized and self confident, with efficient study habits, less time will need to be spent studying, and higher grades will be achieved.

To become self confident, there are many useful steps. The first of these is "self talk." It has been shown through extensive research, that self-talk for students who suffer from test anxiety, should be well monitored, in order to make sure that it contributes to self confidence as opposed to sinking the student. Frequently the self talk of test-anxious students is negative or self-defeating, thinking that everyone else is smarter and faster, that they always mess up, and that if they don't do well, they'll fail the entire course. It is important to decreasing anxiety that awareness is made of self talk. Try writing any negative self thoughts and then disputing them with a positive statement instead. Begin self-encouragement as though it was a friend speaking. Repeat positive statements to help reprogram the mind to believing in successes instead of failures.

Helpful Techniques

Other extremely helpful techniques include:

Self-visualization of doing well and reaching goals
While aiming for an "A" level of understanding, don't try to "overprotect" by setting your expectations lower. This will only convince the mind to stop studying in order to meet the lower expectations.
Don't make comparisons with the results or habits of other students. These are individual factors, and different things work for different people, causing different results.
Strive to become an expert in learning what works well, and what can be done in order to improve. Consider collecting this data in a journal.
Create rewards for after studying instead of doing things before studying that will only turn into avoidance behaviors.
Make a practice of relaxing - by using methods such as progressive relaxation, self-hypnosis, guided imagery, etc - in order to make relaxation an automatic sensation.
Work on creating a state of relaxed concentration so that concentrating will take on the focus of the mind, so that none will be wasted on worrying.
Take good care of the physical self by eating well and getting enough sleep.
Plan in time for exercise and stick to this plan.

Beyond these techniques, there are other methods to be used before, during and after the test that will help the test-taker perform well in addition to overcoming anxiety.

Before the exam comes the academic preparation. This involves establishing a study schedule and beginning at least one week before the actual date of the test. By doing this, the anxiety of not having enough time to study for the test will be automatically eliminated. Moreover, this will make the studying a much more effective experience, ensuring that the learning will be an easier process. This relieves much undue pressure on the test-taker.

Summary sheets, note cards, and flash cards with the main concepts and examples of these main concepts should be prepared in advance of the actual studying time. A topic should never be eliminated from this process. By omitting a topic because it isn't expected to be on the test is only setting up the test-taker for anxiety should it actually appear on the exam. Utilize the course syllabus for laying out the topics that should be studied. Carefully go over the notes that were made in class, paying special attention to any of the issues that the professor took special care to emphasize while lecturing in class. In the textbooks, use the chapter review, or if possible, the chapter tests, to begin your review.

It may even be possible to ask the instructor what information will be covered on the exam, or what the format of the exam will be (for example, multiple choice, essay, free form, true-false). Additionally, see if it is possible to find out how many questions will be on the test. If a review sheet or sample test has been offered by the professor, make good use of it, above anything else, for the preparation for the test. Another great resource for getting to know the examination is reviewing tests from previous semesters. Use these tests to review, and aim to achieve a 100% score on each of the possible topics. With a few exceptions, the goal that you set for yourself is the highest one that you will reach.

Take all of the questions that were assigned as homework, and rework them to any other possible course material. The more problems reworked, the more skill and confidence will form as a result. When forming the solution to a problem, write out each of the steps. Don't simply do head work. By doing as many steps on paper as possible, much clarification and therefore confidence will be formed. Do this with as many homework problems as possible, before checking the answers. By checking the answer after each problem, a reinforcement will exist, that will not be on the exam. Study situations should be as exam-like as possible, to prime the test-taker's system for the experience. By waiting to check the answers at the end, a psychological advantage will be formed, to decrease the stress factor.

Another fantastic reason for not cramming is the avoidance of confusion in concepts, especially when it comes to mathematics. 8-10 hours of study will become one hundred percent more effective if it is spread out over a week or at least several days, instead of doing it all in one sitting. Recognize that the human brain requires time in order to assimilate new material, so frequent breaks and a span of study time over several days will be much more beneficial.

Additionally, don't study right up until the point of the exam. Studying should stop a minimum of one hour before the exam begins. This allows the brain to rest and put things in their proper order. This will also provide the time to become as relaxed as possible when going into the examination room. The test-taker will also have time to eat well and eat sensibly. Know that the brain needs food as much as the rest of the body. With enough food and enough sleep, as well as a relaxed attitude, the body and the mind are primed for success.

Avoid any anxious classmates who are talking about the exam. These students only spread anxiety, and are not worth sharing the anxious sentimentalities.

Before the test also involves creating a positive attitude, so mental preparation should also be a point of concentration. There are many keys to creating a positive attitude. Should fears become rushing in, make a visualization of taking the exam, doing well, and seeing an A written on the paper. Write out a list of affirmations that will bring a feeling of confidence, such as "I am doing well in my English class," "I studied well and know my material," "I enjoy this class." Even if the affirmations aren't believed at first, it sends a positive message to the subconscious which will result in an alteration of the overall belief system, which is the system that creates reality.

If a sensation of panic begins, work with the fear and imagine the very worst! Work through the entire scenario of not passing the test, failing the entire course, and dropping out of school, followed by not getting a job, and pushing a shopping cart through the dark alley where you'll live. This will place things into perspective! Then, practice deep breathing and create a visualization of the opposite situation - achieving an "A" on the exam, passing the entire course, receiving the degree at a graduation ceremony.

On the day of the test, there are many things to be done to ensure the best results, as well as the most calm outlook. The following stages are suggested in order to maximize test-taking potential:

Begin the examination day with a moderate breakfast, and avoid any coffee or beverages with caffeine if the test taker is prone to jitters. Even people who are used to managing caffeine can feel jittery or light-headed when it is taken on a test day.
Attempt to do something that is relaxing before the examination begins. As last minute cramming clouds the mastering of overall concepts, it is better to use this time to create a calming outlook.
Be certain to arrive at the test location well in advance, in order to provide time to select a location that is away from doors, windows and other distractions, as well as giving enough time to relax before the test begins.
Keep away from anxiety generating classmates who will upset the sensation of stability and relaxation that is being attempted before the exam.
Should the waiting period before the exam begins cause anxiety, create a self-distraction by reading a light magazine or something else that is relaxing and simple.

During the exam itself, read the entire exam from beginning to end, and find out how much time should be allotted to each individual problem. Once writing the exam, should more time be taken for a problem, it should be abandoned, in order to begin another problem. If there is time at the end, the unfinished problem can always be returned to and completed.

Read the instructions very carefully - twice - so that unpleasant surprises won't follow during or after the exam has ended.

When writing the exam, pretend that the situation is actually simply the completion of homework within a library, or at home. This will assist in forming a relaxed atmosphere, and will allow the brain extra focus for the complex thinking function.

Begin the exam with all of the questions with which the most confidence is felt. This will build the confidence level regarding the entire exam and will begin a quality momentum. This will also create encouragement for trying the problems where uncertainty resides.

Going with the "gut instinct" is always the way to go when solving a problem. Second guessing should be avoided at all costs. Have confidence in the ability to do well.

For essay questions, create an outline in advance that will keep the mind organized and make certain that all of the points are remembered. For multiple choice, read every answer, even if the correct one has been spotted - a better one may exist.

Continue at a pace that is reasonable and not rushed, in order to be able to work carefully. Provide enough time to go over the answers at the end, to check for small errors that can be corrected.

Should a feeling of panic begin, breathe deeply, and think of the feeling of the body releasing sand through its pores. Visualize a calm, peaceful place, and include all of the sights, sounds and sensations of this image. Continue the deep breathing, and take a few minutes to continue this with closed eyes. When all is well again, return to the test.

If a "blanking" occurs for a certain question, skip it and move on to the next question. There will be time to return to the other question later. Get everything done that can be done, first, to guarantee all the grades that can be compiled, and to build all of the confidence possible. Then return to the weaker questions to build the marks from there.

Remember, one's own reality can be created, so as long as the belief is there, success will follow. And remember: anxiety can happen later, right now, there's an exam to be written!

After the examination is complete, whether there is a feeling for a good grade or a bad grade, don't dwell on the exam, and be certain to follow through on the reward that was promised...and enjoy it! Don't dwell on any mistakes that have been made, as there is nothing that can be done at this point anyway.

Additionally, don't begin to study for the next test right away. Do something relaxing for a while, and let the mind relax and prepare itself to begin absorbing information again.

From the results of the exam - both the grade and the entire experience, be certain to learn from what has gone on. Perfect studying habits and work some more on confidence in order to make the next examination experience even better than the last one.

Learn to avoid places where openings occurred for laziness, procrastination and day dreaming.

Use the time between this exam and the next one to better learn to relax, even learning to relax on cue, so that any anxiety can be controlled during the next exam. Learn how to relax the body. Slouch in your chair if that helps. Tighten and then relax all of the different muscle groups, one group at a time, beginning with the feet and then working all the way up to the neck and face. This will ultimately relax the muscles more than they were to begin with. Learn how to breathe deeply and comfortably, and focus on this breathing going in and out as a relaxing thought. With every exhale, repeat the word "relax."

As common as test anxiety is, it is very possible to overcome it. Make yourself one of the test-takers who overcome this frustrating hindrance.

Additional Bonus Material

Due to our efforts to try to keep this book to a manageable length, we've created a link that will give you access to all of your additional bonus material.

Please visit http://www.mometrix.com/bonus948/cnn to access the information.